T0059817

A Field Guide to Men's Health

ARTISAN
NEW YORK

A Field Guide to Men's Health

Eat Right, Stay Fit, Sleep Well, and Have Great Sex— Forever

Jesse N. Mills, MD
with Will Cockrell

Copyright © 2021 by Jesse N. Mills, MD
Illustrations copyright © 2021 by Jason Pickersgill, except for pages 60 and 199, copyright © 2021 by Shutterstock Inc./Double Brain

Library of Congress Cataloging-in-Publication Data

Names: Mills, Jesse N., author.
Title: A field guide to men's health : eat right, stay fit, sleep well, and have great sex—forever / Jesse N. Mills, MD.
Description: New York, NY : Artisan, a division of Workman Publishing Co., Inc., 2021. | Includes index.
Identifiers: LCCN 2021014416 | ISBN 9781579659783 (paperback)
Subjects: LCSH: Men—Health and hygiene. | Self-care, Health.
Classification: LCC RA777.8 .M56 2021 | DDC 613/.04234—dc23
LC record available at https://lccn.loc.gov/2021014416

Design by Suet Chong

Artisan books are available at special discounts when purchased in bulk for premiums and sales promotions as well as for fund-raising or educational use. Special editions or book excerpts also can be created to specification. For details, contact the Special Sales Director at the address below, or send an e-mail to specialmarkets@workman.com.

For speaking engagements, contact speakersbureau@workman.com.

Published by Artisan
A division of Workman Publishing Co., Inc.
225 Varick Street
New York, NY 10014-4381
artisanbooks.com

Artisan is a registered trademark of Workman Publishing Co., Inc.

Published simultaneously in Canada by Thomas Allen & Son, Limited

Printed in China

First printing, November 2021

10 9 8 7 6 5 4 3 2 1

For KMM:MNP forever.

You are my everything.

CONTENTS

I'M GLAD YOU'RE HERE

Ever notice how a guy won't go to the doctor unless his arm or his penis is broken? It's true, men are far less likely than women to take care of themselves and see their doctors regularly. Men are even less likely to *have* a regular doctor. Part of a guy's reluctance to see a physician stems from the mixed signals he gets from the media about his health. It's hard not to be confused when one study says drinking alcohol or coffee is bad for us and another says it's good; or when we're told sugar is the enemy, but that artificial sweetener will make us fatter, or even kill us.

Men may have less genetic information than women do, but we are still incredibly complex creatures. And when it comes to health, one size does not fit all. In fact, men today are more diverse than ever. Take a look at a college or high school class photo from the late nineteenth century, when obesity was rare in the United States. All the men in that sepia-faded image will be lean, but none will be muscle bound. A class photo from the 1950s will show that men became a bit thicker, as processed foods became more ubiquitous after World War II. Now look at the class of 2000 or 2020 and you'll see a mix of a few skinny guys, a lot more overweight guys, and a few buff guys: a bell curve of weight distribution in the modern male.

So what's changed in a hundred years? We've learned a ton about exercise, nutrition, and managing diseases. And with knowledge came confusion. More data has actually led to *less* understanding. The multibillion-dollar wellness industry encourages us to believe we can buy change in a bottle. But men's wellness is more about clever marketing—instead of yoga, it's *brog*a, Botox is *Brotox*—than a holistic approach. I don't even know what "wellness" means, and yet it's something I'm supposed to aspire to. For many men, trying to achieve today's ideals has led to stress, disappointment, and, ultimately, a lot of dudes just giving up. And giving up is exactly what leads us to looking and feeling like that unhealthy guy in the middle of the bell curve. We jump on the latest diet craze and quickly drop 20 pounds, then gain it all back even quicker.

This book will pull back the curtain and simplify things. My goal is for you to realize that feeling great is not that complicated. Let's do away with the hype. Let's take a deep breath and figure out how to optimize your general health and, yes, your *sexual* health. It's not that hard.

That said, I do believe three basic rules are universal: eat less, move more, and sleep better. These are rules you can riff on for the rest of your life. They provide a guide to optimizing your time on earth. Men's health is cardiovascular health, mental health, sexual health, lifestyle, and nutrition. It's about understanding exercise, moderation, and the importance of sleep and healthy relationships. And yes, it's about having a healthy penis. This is a book to empower you to take charge of your life, to help you find a health professional ally to manage the medical aspects, and for you to take accountability for your own well-being.

We'll learn about the basics of nutrition and the differences among carbs, fat, and protein, as well as why people tend to complicate things when they're trying to eat well. We'll learn about exercise, and about the difference between cardio and strength training. We'll learn that washboard abs are an unrealistic goal for most men. I'll talk about finding a healthcare provider who is familiar with *all* aspects of men's health. We'll look at handling stress, too. Stress kills. It's bad for your heart, bad for sleep, bad for sex. We have to get a handle on stress and find activities and people that *de*stress us. I don't have a cure for stress—I suffer from it just as much as you do. But I hope to help you learn how to deal with stress positively.

This is a book for *all* adult men, from 20-year-olds to 100-year-olds, for the former college athlete who needs to get back into shape and for the heavier guy who is feeling ashamed and hopeless. It's for a guy on multiple medications for high cholesterol, high blood pressure, and diabetes, looking to change the habits that got him there in the first place. These men will have different journeys ahead of them. And that's totally cool.

Open this book to a section, read it, and if it resonates, make that one small change to better your life. I want to empower you to decide what advice is right for you.

This book, like life, spends a lot of time in gray areas. I don't believe in a world with only two pathways. Better health isn't all in or all out. Men are much more complicated; some days, some weeks, we bring it and some days, some weeks, we're too beat down. Just don't let those beat-down days or weeks turn to months or years. Above all else, I want to emphasize the importance of embracing who we are. No more judgment—don't shame the out-of-shape guy, the skinny guy, or the superbuff guy—let's all just be us. Then ask yourself: How do you want to *look*? How do you want to *feel*? How do you want to *live*? By honestly answering these three simple questions, you've taken the first—and perhaps most important—step in *your* journey.

Why should you listen to me?

My understanding of—and enthusiasm for—a holistic approach to men's health is both professional and personal. I went to medical school to become a surgeon—a microsurgeon, to be specific. (I sew together the tiniest parts of the male reproductive system, like the vas deferens, epididymis, and the blood vessels circulating in the testicles.) I love working with my hands, identifying a problem, and fixing it. I'm a urologist, which means I'm trained to treat everything from prostate cancer to kidney stones to erectile dysfunction. But as a urologist, I also see myself as a general men's health doctor for the very reason that men don't typically go to the doctor unless they have a urologic problem. Many of my patients don't have primary-care physicians, so I'm the one who ends up getting them on the right path to healthier living and making sure they have excellent primary care to round out their healthcare team. My enthusiasm for empowering men to lead a healthy, inspired life spurred me to found a comprehensive men's health center in Colorado in 2013. Two years later, I took this knowledge and came to UCLA to establish the Men's Clinic at UCLA.

I am also a father of two nearly grown boys. As a father and husband, I'm keenly aware of my own responsibility to take care of myself. I am constantly applying my own unique perspective as a physician, surgeon, and infertility specialist to my own health, as well as to help my patients live better. I practice what I teach, but I also love life. Life is food, sometimes rich food. Life is an occasional glass of wine or a cocktail. We *can* live a healthy, fit, and long life even if we hit it hard every once in a while. I believe in exercising—heavy, sweaty exercise—four days a week or more, but also in indulging one or two days a week. I like cheat days—though I prefer to call them reward days (see page 100)—so long as you have your nutrition in order every other day of the week.

I don't preach to my patients. I dialogue: I tell the men who see me in my office that we'll be spending only about 45 minutes a year together, so the remaining 364 days, 23 hours, and 15 minutes are up to them. I coach men to invest in their health. It's time for me to bring these years of experience and professing to a book everyone can read—a book for men *and* the men and women they're partnered with.

This is not a shortcut. Nor do I have all the answers. But I have made it my mission to cut through the noise and give men something they can really use. For some, it will start a conversation; for others, it may save a life. This is a book for them— and every man in between.

01

RESET

A Man's Guide to the Basics

The good news is better living is all basic. Why do you need a reset? Because you're overwhelmed. Every time you click on a link about the newest diet fad or the best new exercise that will make you live longer, you're confused. Why does it have to be so hard? It doesn't. Good, solid advice to optimize a man's health is easy. Applying this advice will take some work on your part; you'll need to assemble a team, and you'll need an open mind. Your team will be your family, friends and at least one healthcare provider. If you have chronic medical problems such as heart disease, diabetes, kidney problems, you're going to need a bigger team.

Finding the Right Medical Team

If you don't have a doctor, it's time to get one. If you do have a doctor, it's time to start asking more questions and take control of your health. **A great doctor will help you understand the value of being *proactive* instead of *reactive* when it comes to your health.** Great doctors don't just fix things, they help you develop habits that keep you off medications for as long as possible, keep you out of an operating room, and, in many cases, keep serious stuff from becoming *too* serious. I can't overstate the value of having an internist or a family physician who can get to know you. Take the time and effort to find someone you trust and can stick with.

FINDING A GREAT DOCTOR

First and foremost, you need a good primary-care provider: either a physician (an internist or general practitioner), physician assistant, or nurse practitioner. This needs to be someone who is knowledgeable in preventive medicine—an expert in how to stay *out* of the doctor's office. Ideally, your primary-care provider should have at least an interest in specific men's health topics, such as sexual dysfunction. The best way to find a great doctor is to do a little research, ask a friend or colleague for a recommendation, and make an appointment—if the practitioner doesn't fit your personality or share your health values, move on.

When starting from scratch, begin with the three A's:

- **Able.** Your doc needs to be good at what she or he does and have graduated from a respected medical school, though it doesn't necessarily have to be a top-ten school. (There are plenty of not-so-good docs from great schools and plenty of fantastic physicians from lower-tier schools; don't bask in the pedigree too much.) Your physicians should also be board certified, meaning they have taken qualifying exams in their specialty and are recognized by their peers as qualified to treat patients at the highest level.

- **Available.** Your doc should see you in a reasonable amount of time and respect your time so you're not in the waiting room too long.

- **Affable.** Your doc should be nice. Your time is valuable, and your concerns are valuable—don't settle for a dismissive physician. Medical schools have recently invested a lot of time training future physicians to be more compassionate. You should seek out a doctor who truly cares about you.

MDs Versus DOs

Physicians either graduate from medical doctor (MD) schools or doctor of osteopathic medicine (DO) schools. There is no functional difference between an MD and a DO physician—both practice medicine, both can perform surgery. The difference is philosophical and historical. Doctors of osteopathic medicine focus a little more on holistic practice and are trained to incorporate musculoskeletal alignment into their practices.

When You Need a Specialist

Perhaps you have a condition that requires a more specialized touch. A urologist like myself, for example, will lead the way for any sexual health, fertility, or testosterone issues. But it's important you find a urologist who specializes in *men's* health. Check prospective doctors' web pages to determine if they did a fellowship (extra training) in sexual medicine or infertility. See if they belong to infertility or sexual medicine societies such as the Sexual Medicine Society of North America, the American Society for Reproductive Medicine, or the American Society for Men's Health. These are great indicators of a deep understanding of male-specific issues.

What If Your Doctor Tries to Sell You Products?

Don't be immediately turned off by a physician with a side hustle. Medical professionals have seen major declines in salary, more than most other industries. Over the past 20 years, physician reimbursements from insurance companies and national and state governmental agencies have dropped dramatically. Meanwhile, overhead to run a medical practice has skyrocketed. This is why most physicians see many more patients than the previous generation and why very few independent solo practices exist. This has also spurred a lot of physicians to sell products directly to patients. If you're seeing a dermatologist, for example, he or she may suggest you buy the practice's proprietary sunscreen. If you're seeing a wellness physician, you may be offered supplements or medical devices to improve your response to the therapy. Is that bad? I guess it depends. Investigate the product and price-shop. But always walk away from the *hard* sell—that's never cool.

Ignore Online Reviews

When looking for a doctor, *please* ignore online reviews. These are often bogus and are not vetted in any way. They typically relay horror stories that say very little about the quality of a doctor's care. And it goes both ways—both glowing five-star reviews and scathing one-star reviews are equally unhelpful. By the same token, avoid doctors who advertise that they are the *world's foremost expert* in anything. There is no governing world expert board, no Super Bowl ring for doctors. I get weekly junk email from multiple sources telling me I'm the best doctor in America, and for $500, I can send away for a plaque to proudly display in my waiting room. C'mon. Buying into this will land you in the office of practitioners who care more about their image than your care. If the doctors have a website, look for a list of articles and publications they have written or contributed to; this gives you an idea of a physician's area of expertise.

Paging Dr. Web

I have no problem with my patients looking up their symptoms, shopping for doctors, and getting as much advice online as they can before they see me. If you're reading material from respected medical institutions, written by specialists in the field, you're probably okay. For example, sites like WebMD and those of medical institutions like the Mayo Clinic, Cleveland Clinic, or UCLA (my particular favorite) can be great sources of high-quality medical information and advice. Understand that a lot of the content is outdated, but it's not dangerous, and it's a solid starting point for a conversation with your doctor at your next appointment. And a lot of good comes from online medical communities, such as kidney donor chains or support networks for medical conditions from diabetes to dementia.

However, getting medical advice *solely* from online sources can be catastrophic, as the medical myths and snake oils perpetuated online are nothing short of disgusting. The whole antivaccination movement, for example, would not have taken off quite like it did if not for the internet. There is nothing worse for us doctors than when a patient develops false ideas that we have to dispel in order to deliver the best care we can. So how do you know if something you read online is legit? First, if the source is trying to sell you something, don't buy it until you check with your doctor. If the product or program sounds too good to be true, it is likely a hoax.

Believe it or not, some people out there try to sell us totally unproven, sometimes dangerous treatments for pandemics. I wish it were criminal, and this practice goes back centuries. I've seen ads for drinking silver solutions as a cure for COVID-19. There is no proof this does anything other than cost a lot of money and prevent sick people from getting actual medical care. Bottom line: if someone is trying to sell you something to cure a virus, stay away, check with your trusted health professional, or do a little online research from better sources. The internet health marketplace is nothing more than a high-tech traveling medicine show.

HEALTH BY THE DECADES

Once your pediatrician stops giving you cartoon Band-Aids and kicks you out of the office because you no longer fit on the exam table, what do you do? As you can imagine, the younger you are, the fewer well-man checkups you need. Let's break it down by age.

20s to 30s

If you're doing what I ask of you in this book, you shouldn't need more than an annual checkup with a primary-care provider. At your annual physical evaluation, your doctor will check vital signs, order a blood test to determine cholesterol levels, and perform a urine test. Based on any symptoms you express, your physician may also order blood sugar levels, testosterone levels, inflammatory markers like C-Reactive Protein, and possibly thyroid levels.

40s

The checkup doesn't change much: you still need a vitals check, a cholesterol check, and a urine test. If you have a family history of cancers such as prostate or colon, your primary doc may suggest screening for these diseases now, whereas no family history means you can wait until you turn 45.

50s

If you've developed some health conditions, perhaps diabetes, heart or kidney disease, or obesity, your primary physician may refer you to specialists to help manage these chronic issues. At 45, it's time for your first colonoscopy, so you'll need to find a gastroenterologist for that procedure. As a urologist, I have a bias that men should check in with me around age 50. That's not necessary if your primary doc is comfortable managing any prostate or sexual issues you start developing by then, but your primary has a lot of stuff to manage and may not have the time to do a deeper dive into your urinary and sexual habits. And as we'll learn in the prostate health section (see page 66), prostate cancer screening is complicated and controversial. It may be good to have an expert opinion.

60s and Beyond

Annual checkups will get a little more involved and will depend on what health baggage you've accumulated along your journey.

A CALL TO ACTION Don't wait for something to go wrong before you seek out a doctor. It can take weeks to months to get an appointment with a good, busy physician. If you already have something going on and you call for an appointment, you may not get in as quickly as you need. Once you've secured an appointment, prepare for that first visit by writing down any specific questions you have. A good physician should ask you what the most pressing concerns are, but they only have so much time in a standard 20-minute visit. Lastly, you have to feel comfortable with your physician. If you don't, no harm in changing docs.

YOUR MEDICAL TEAM

Many men don't see a doctor as regularly as they should because they simply don't know which doctor does what and where to begin. Here is all you need to know to take action today to assemble an all-star men's health team.

DOCTOR	ROLE
Family doctor	A family practice physician has general medical training in pediatric and adult medicine and often practices in rural areas. Some specialize in sports medicine.
Internist	An internist is important from age 20 on, but the older you get, the more crucial this doc becomes. An internist goes a little more in depth than a family doc and can diagnose and treat common chronic medical conditions, such as diabetes, high cholesterol, and high blood pressure.
Cardiologist	Heart specialists are not typically necessary until after age 50 unless—and it's a big *unless*—you have early heart issues.
Endocrinologist	Endocrinologists specialize in diagnosing and treating hormone disorders such as thyroid issues, diabetes, or testosterone imbalances. Your internist will typically spot the issue and refer you.

DOCTOR	ROLE
Urologist	Urologists deal with sexual function, urinary function, prostate issues, and testosterone therapy. While any man with any of these issues should see a urologist, these are issues that are more common in men over 50.
Gastroenterologist	Once a man hits 45, he'll need a gastroenterologist to perform a colonoscopy. A GI can also help men suffering from inflammatory bowel disease, chronic constipation, diarrhea, or any other malady of the intestinal tract.
Dermatologist	Dermatologists screen and treat skin cancer, and cosmetic dermatologists can administer Botox or fillers to improve a man's appearance.
Mental health professional	From psychiatrists to psychologists to social workers to sex therapists, mental health professionals are an important part of a men's health team. Men suffering from depression will benefit from psychiatric evaluation and talking with a therapist. Men with all sorts of sexual dysfunction can get a lot out of speaking with a sex therapist.

They're Called Vitals for a Reason

In many ways, the vast majority of information and advice in this book is in service of the most important organ in your body: your heart. Everything from the food you eat to the amount of sleep you get to your stress levels will affect heart function. Frankly, if your heart isn't working right, not much else matters until it does. But the good news is that the situation works the other way around, too: live well, and heart health will likely follow.

IT ALL STARTS WITH A HEALTHY HEART

Heart disease is the leading killer for *all* humans. Men do not have more heart problems than women. So whether you're male or female, take incredibly good care of your heart. And almost anything you do to improve heart health will improve your sexual health. Here's what you need to know.

Cholesterol: Know Your Numbers

It's so important to understand the difference between your HDL ("good" cholesterol) and LDL ("bad" cholesterol) because these numbers are highly individual. Cholesterol itself is not *bad*, per se. It's kind of like salt: our bodies need cholesterol. Our brains need cholesterol to function properly, our endocrine system needs cholesterol to make hormones. All dietary cholesterol comes from animal sources, but that doesn't mean men who avoid meat or dairy have low cholesterol levels. In fact, our bodies make cholesterol, which is why someone who eats a vegan diet can have high cholesterol levels. But some people's bodies generate way more cholesterol than they need, and high cholesterol often indicates an increased risk of serious heart disease. Know your numbers and know your risk factors. If you have close blood relatives who developed heart disease in their early 60s or younger, you have to be careful and may need to go on a cholesterol-reducing drug, known as a statin. Statins save lives: the medical literature is clear on this. However, statins have a lot of side effects, including muscle weakness or even painful muscle breakdown, possible liver and kidney damage, and a host of other issues. The best advice is to try to avoid statins, but for men with a history of heart attack, it's a choice between statin side effects or another heart attack. Following a strict heart-healthy diet, like the one popularized by Dr. Dean Ornish in the 1980s, may allow you to avoid taking a statin. We'll discuss the Ornish diet in chapter 3 (see page 85), but essentially, it's a super-low-fat, high-fiber diet—no meat or fatty dairy; lots of fresh veggies, whole grains, and fruit. It is supported by great scientific data, but the diet is not easy to stick to. Also be mindful that exercise is excellent for reducing cholesterol.

The Most *Vital* Vital Sign: Blood Pressure

Sadly, high blood pressure (hypertension) still claims a lot of men's lives. High blood pressure increases your risk of heart attack, stroke, kidney failure, and—oh yeah—erectile dysfunction. If you don't care about your kidneys, at least look after your heart for the sake of your penis. **Guys should check their blood pressure every couple of months, easily done with an inexpensive, reliable home blood pressure monitor available from local big-box stores, drugstores, or online vendors.** Expect to pay $35 to $50 for a good one—they last for years. **Keeping your blood pressure under control can be achieved by doing all the things we talk about in this book: eat well, move more, and sleep better.** There is a reason blood pressure is one of the vital signs: it's vital to your health, longevity, and happiness. But some men develop hypertension despite a perfect lifestyle. These men should take blood pressure lowering medicine, as it can save their hearts, kidneys, and livers.

Your Heart Rate

This is an important baseline for tracking heart health as well as calculating optimal exercise effort. The better shape you're in, the lower your resting heart rate is and the higher your exercise heart rate (see page 130) can get. For men in reasonable shape, resting heart rates should be in the range of 65 to 80 beats per minute. If you're an endurance athlete in great shape, your resting heart rate could be in the 40s—that's okay; your heart is so efficient, it doesn't need to beat as often to supply your resting body with oxygen-rich blood. Home blood pressure monitors or fitness heart rate monitors are the most accurate way to read your heart rate, but there are several, albeit less accurate, DIY options.

Carotid pulse   Take two fingers and drag them down from your jawbone until they are one finger-width below the jawbone and one or two finger-widths up from your windpipe. Press lightly and you should feel your pulse. Look at your watch or timer, count how many pulses you feel in 30 seconds, and multiply that number by 2.

Radial pulse   Turn your wrist so your palm faces skyward. Take two fingers of other hand and lightly drag them from the fleshy part of your hand at the base of your thumb. About two finger-widths below your hand, you will feel your pulse. Look at your watch or timer, count how many pulses you feel in 30 seconds, and multiply that number by 2.

OTHER RED FLAGS THAT CANNOT BE IGNORED

Aside from our vital signs, there are a few more telltale clues that something may be seriously wrong. **Bleeding from any orifice is almost always bad.** With the exception of the occasional bloody nose, if you're experiencing any of the following, see your doctor immediately and request a full workup. Denial is powerful. I've had male patients who urinated blood for months to years before they came in for an evaluation. Since blood in the urine can be a warning sign of bladder or kidney cancer, that's a bad idea. As with all things in medicine, early detection is key to the best prognosis.

Coughing blood. This could be a sign of lung cancer, tuberculosis, bleeding from the stomach or esophagus, or other inflammatory condition of the lung. There is no home remedy for coughing blood. If you're doing this, call your doctor today or tomorrow to get worked up.

Blood in your stool. This could be a few things. If you're under age 45, it may be hemorrhoids. If you're 45 and haven't had a colonoscopy yet, it's time, as the bleeding could be a sign of cancer (even if you're under 45). If it's bright, copious blood, the problem is likely in the colon, the last part of the intestinal tract. If the blood is dark and tarry, the problem could be in the stomach. It's important to get checked by your doctor as soon as you can. Inflammatory bowel diseases such as Crohn's disease and ulcerative colitis can also cause intestinal bleeding and need evaluation by a gastroenterologist.

Blood in your urine. This could be from the kidneys, the ureter (the tube connecting the kidney to the bladder), the bladder, the prostate, or the urethra (the channel that connects the bladder to the penis). See a urologist right away. To diagnose the source of the blood, your urologist will order a CT scan and schedule you for a cystoscopy. She or he will use a cystoscope— a long, skinny, and flexible tube camera—to look at the urethra, prostate, and bladder. The urologist may also order urine tests looking for cancer cells. One possible source of the bleeding is kidney and bladder stones. And men with big prostates can bleed into the urine as well. If you smoke cigarettes and have blood in your urine, there's a chance you have cancer of the bladder or kidney. Smokers have a much higher risk of bladder cancer than nonsmokers. The good news is, the quicker a smoker gets evaluated, the more likely he'll have a good outcome.

Ejaculating blood. Surprisingly, this isn't usually too serious. Most likely you haven't ejaculated in a while, and a forceful orgasm simply ruptured a blood vessel in the prostate—it'll heal in a few days. But still let your doc know! Blood in the semen (hematospermia) can look bright red, can appear as streaks of blood within the normal pearly semen color, or can appear rusty. Usually a man ejaculates and notices red streaks or drops of blood in the semen. Subsequent ejaculations take on a rusty color as the ruptured blood vessel heals. Persistent hematospermia, lasting over weeks or months, can be from a prostate infection, stones in the prostate, or, rarely, prostate cancer. It's an easy checkup with a urologist to find the source and, usually, be reassured.

SEE A DOCTOR IMMEDIATELY IF . . .
You Have Chest Pain

Heart disease presents differently in men than in women. Men tend to develop heart disease about ten years sooner, and are usually more symptomatic. Men also get chest pain frequently as a sign of a pending heart attack. **Chest pain is a heart attack until the emergency room tells you otherwise.** This is especially true if the pain comes when you are more physically active than usual. Say you haven't gone jogging in a while, but you feel inspired to hit the track. A quarter mile in, you're clutching your chest—call 911 as you fall to the pitch. **Men under age 60 with chest pain tend to die more often than men over 60 because the heart hasn't had time to make new blood vessels to bypass the blocked ones.** It's critical to always check with your doctor before starting a physical fitness program.

MARIO, 44

Pressure Drop

Mario was 44 when I met him. He is an attorney in a high-stress law firm and came to me after experiencing difficulty getting erections. He was a college football player, admits that he gained a few pounds and wasn't exercising as much as he used to. He didn't have a primary physician—came to me because he found my profile as a sexual medicine specialist online and didn't want to "waste" his time with a primary doc if I could treat him. Before I even walked in the room to greet him, I saw his vital signs: blood pressure was 180/110, which is critically elevated! After interviewing him, I learned his father had a stroke when he was 38, his mom has diabetes and is obese, and he has an older brother with prostate cancer diagnosed when he was 51. I let Mario know I was delighted to treat his erections but we both had some work to do. He needed a primary physician to manage his blood pressure and evaluate his risk of stroke (spoiler alert—high blood pressure equals a huge risk for stroke) and diabetes. Mario's erectile problem was his wake-up call that he needed to get serious about his health. When I saw him three months later, he had lost 10 pounds by eating leaner meals and exercising more, and his blood pressure returned to normal with a low-dose blood pressure pill and his lifestyle changes. As a Black man, statistically, Mario is more at risk for developing prostate cancer earlier than a white man. I screened him for prostate cancer and reassured him he was fine for now but that he needs to get checked every year. With Mario's newfound motivation, the expert care of his new primary physician, and my guidance, not only did Mario get his erections back, but he also decreased his risk of suffering a stroke, developing diabetes, and having undiagnosed prostate cancer.

Building a Superhuman Immune System

Getting sick sucks, right? Even a common cold can—and should—keep you out of the office and feeling crummy for a few days. Then there's the flu, which can make you miserable for a week or more and can be dangerous. So how do you avoid getting sick? Before we discuss pills, let's make it simpler. The best tool to prevent illness is to *avoid* illness.

THE NEW NORMAL

With the coronavirus pandemic of 2020, the world learned a lot about sickness and contagion. As I write this book, there is no cure, and people are still dying at an alarming rate in some countries. This pandemic will pass, as have all plagues over the course of human civilization. And we have a vaccine. What we do know is that once COVID-19 ceases to kill hundreds of people daily, a new pandemic will eventually arise. Fortunately, there are things a guy can do to keep himself and his family safe and prepared now and in the future. Let's briefly explore what our immune system is and what it does so we can learn to make it stronger.

The world is full of microscopic organisms that do everything from proofing bread and fermenting beer to causing pandemics. Over the millennia, our bodies have adapted to our environments and lived harmoniously with millions of these microorganisms—good bacteria keep our guts healthy just as good yeast raises our bread. But bad microorganisms are out there as well. Always have been. So we build defenses. Our skin is our biggest immune organ. For example, tetanus is a deadly bacteria that lives in the ground. You can step on the tetanus bacteria all you want, and it won't hurt you. But if you step on a nail in the dirt and puncture your skin, you could die from tetanus—if you weren't vaccinated.

Because we have to eat, breathe, see, hear, procreate, urinate, and defecate, we have to have holes in our skin. Therefore, we have a beautiful complex system of internal defenses to protect ourselves from invaders that get in through all of our orifices. These defense systems are cells and proteins your body has to make. **Strengthen your immune system by taking better care of yourself. Stay true to the pillars of this book: eat, move, sleep.**

Prepping for the Next Pandemic

Pandemics aside, many of my overall philosophies about staying healthy will serve you well in keeping your immune system in top form. Do you catch every cold that comes through the office? What about the flu? Get your flu shot every year— immunization is not perfect, and you can still get the flu, but your chances of a severe case go way down. If you find yourself prone to colds, first thing you do is wash your hands more often. Carry hand sanitizer in your car and stock it at your desk, then use it. Cold viruses linger on surfaces, so don't touch your face, nose, or mouth without washing or sanitizing your hands first. **Men with chronic disease get sicker more frequently than men who are fit and who exercise more and sleep well.** COVID-19 preys most heavily on men with other diseases. In fact, a man with one chronic illness—say a history of lung disease, diabetes, obesity, or heart disease—has a ten times higher risk of dying from the infection. So think of boosting your immunity as preparing for the next pandemic: lose weight, control your blood sugars, exercise vigorously at least three to five days a week, and sleep a solid six to eight hours. Do these things and not only will you get fewer colds, your risk of dying from any infectious disease drops significantly.

Our Socially Distant Society

Humans are social. We thrive on connections, and the COVID-19 pandemic fundamentally altered our view of social gatherings. As the world opens up postpandemic, consider where you want to be exposed. Is going to a movie theater or gym ever a good idea anymore? Or being in a crowded bar, restaurant, or concert worth the exposure? You have to personally decide the risk you are willing to take, knowing that science sees that the fewer close interactions you have with people, the lower your risk of contracting a respiratory or direct-contact disease.

That said, protecting yourself doesn't necessarily mean staying put. Say you can't hole up in an isolated compound. Say you have to work around other people and make a living. A bunch of nonmedical commonsense measures greatly reduced transmission of COVID-19 and likely will work for any new airborne-spread virus. **Simple physical distancing works:** you can't catch something from someone if the virus can't hop from one host to the next. **Hand washing works:** if you touch something an infected person has touched, and you touch your mouth, eyes, nose, or wherever before washing your hands, you've transmitted the virus to yourself. If the virus figures out how to get past your skin or mucous membranes, you now have the illness.

Vaccinations Work. Period.

Get vaccinated! Here's a philosophical observation: up until the coronavirus pandemic of 2020, the United States had not seen a devastating infectious disease that was so easily transmissible to millions of citizens since polio. My parents witnessed their friends die from polio. Their friends who survived polio and are alive today still have limps or persistent disability from this horrible disease. You would be hard pressed to find Americans in their 70s who are antivaccine. But if you've never seen a friend die of polio, but you've seen people with vaccination reactions, you might think *polio can't be so bad*. I predict that once we implement the vaccine for coronavirus that allows the world to return to some state of normalcy, people of all ages will start believing in vaccines again. Some people are at risk for vaccine side effects; the rest of us are unlikely to experience anything serious. Ultimately it's a risk worth taking for the benefit of a healthy society.

THE IMPORTANCE OF HAND WASHING

Doctors first realized hand washing prevented infection in the mid-1800s. Hungarian physician Ignaz Semmelweis observed that when doctors delivered babies after performing autopsies, there was a higher maternal death rate than when midwives delivered babies. He hypothesized that doctors were transmitting something from the cadavers to the women in labor (remember, this was before we knew what bacteria were). So Semmelweis forced all of the doctors in his hospital to wash their hands with chlorine lime before they delivered babies and he saw a dramatic drop in maternal death from infection. It took many more years to identify the bacterium that was responsible for maternal mortality in childbirth, but the scientific community owes a lot to Dr. Semmelweis. Simple hand washing is one of the greatest weapons in reducing the spread of all infections. Always wash your hands before you touch your face. If you touch a door handle, then scratch your nose or rub your eyes, you've just wiped onto yourself whatever the last hundred people who touched that door handle had on their hands. Yuck!

OVER-THE-COUNTER IMMUNE BOOSTERS

While a lot of supplements are touted to boost immunity, there are only three things that might be worth a try.

Vitamin C

Humans, some other primates, and guinea pigs are the only mammals that can't make vitamin C. Vitamin C helps produce collagen. It's crucial for gum health and wound healing and, at normal doses, is essential to prevent scurvy (something you've probably never heard of unless you read maritime history). About 50 years ago, Linus Pauling, a two-time Nobel Laureate, became convinced that high-dose vitamin C was the best treatment to boost the immune system, prevent cancer, and decrease the risk of getting viruses. He personally took 5 grams a day and researched the supplement exhaustively until he passed away (well into his 90s). But he produced little data. To this day, no one has shown that vitamin C does much of anything when you megadose. But it also does not appear to be toxic, so you're welcome to take it.

Dosing of 250 milligrams a day is plenty to boost your immunity. There are some studies showing vitamin C at 500 milligrams a day can improve your fertility. For men trying to initiate a pregnancy, I recommend 500 milligrams a day of a high-quality supplement. If you want to get your vitamin C naturally, eat more citrus—squeeze a lime or lemon into your water. Eat a couple of clementines a day. Peppers and broccoli are also great sources of vitamin C. Cut up a raw red bell pepper, toss it in your salad, and you're all set.

Zinc

The mineral zinc is found in many over-the-counter cold supplements. Despite a lot of research, there's little science proving its effectiveness. One recent meta-analysis, the sketchiest of scientific studies, concluded that 75 milligrams a day of zinc *may* decrease the duration of the common cold by 30 percent—and that's not bad for a harmless supplement. Stick to that reasonable dose and see if it works for you.

Vitamin D

Vitamin D is incredibly important. Actually, it's a hormone that strengthens bone. Children with low vitamin D levels can develop a deforming bone condition called rickets—fortunately very rare in developed countries these days because vitamin D is added to dietary staples like milk, bread, and cereals. Symptoms of vitamin D deficiency are vague: bone and muscle ache, fatigue, low mood—none of which you want. So how do you get enough vitamin D, and how does it affect your immune system?

We know sunshine exposure stimulates natural production of this essential hormone. We know vitamin D is important to bone health. And that men with higher vitamin D levels have a healthier immune system, but megadosing with vitamin D supplements—we just don't have great data. However, getting a little sun exposure every day is good for your natural vitamin D levels and good for maintaining mood, and that's an immune booster right there. You don't need more than fifteen minutes a day of sunlight on any exposed skin to up your vitamin D levels.

Vitamin D improves your bone density—but not as much as weight-bearing exercise. If you wish to start a vitamin D supplement, 2,000 units a day is a good place to begin. If you aren't lucky enough to live in a sunny, warm climate year-round, supplementing with vitamin D is important in wintertime.

DON'T OVERUSE ANTIBIOTICS

It may sound strange, but one of the best ways to boost your immune system is to avoid antibiotics. Frequent antibiotic use depletes your natural immune system and sets you up for more serious infections. We've arrived at a time in medicine where we physicians realize that we can't rely on antibiotics to treat every ear, respiratory, or gut infection, as the bacteria have become smarter—they've figured out how to become resistant to antibiotics and thus wreak havoc on humankind. You have to take responsibility for antibiotic use as well. Some men are upset that I won't prescribe antibiotics unless there are clear signs of an infection. Once I explain to the guy that I'm doing him a favor, he usually understands. But many physicians feel pressure to prescribe. Save the antibiotic for when you're really sick.

THE IMPORTANCE OF GUT HEALTH

There's nothing like a healthy bowel evacuation first thing in the morning: it's a sign of good health and a great day ahead. Maybe I feel this way because I'm getting older—older guys appreciate this sort of thing; younger guys, well, if you're lucky enough, you'll get there sooner than you want or think. Regularity is a sign of a balanced diet and healthy stress levels. Consult a physician if you chronically have diarrhea, constipation, or any irregularity in your bowel movements; you may have an inflammatory bowel disorder. Inflammatory bowel and irritable bowel disease are poorly understood phenomena that cause significant discomfort, lost work hours, and anxiety. There are many potential causes for inflammatory bowel disorders, including pathological bacteria and autoimmune disorders. But the common thread to poor bowel regularity is stress. I can't overemphasize the importance of stress reduction here. You may even benefit from breathing exercises and meditation to improve your stressed-out bowels.

Not Going on the Regular?

Here are a few ways to get things moving.

Eat more fiber. Fiber fuels good digestion and is found in stringy vegetables like kale and chard and in whole grains with husks (used in some breads).

The Pros and Cons of Probiotics

Probiotics sound great. Our lower intestines are lined with colonies of healthy bacteria to aid in digestion, boost our immunity, and keep the bad bacteria out (in fact, when you take an antibiotic, one of the most common side effects is diarrhea because you just killed off your good bacteria). It would seem to make sense, then, that swallowing new, healthy bacteria will restore your natural gut health. The problem is, whatever you take in your mouth goes through your whole digestive tract before it ends up in your colon, and when a probiotic hits your stomach, your stomach acids destroy nearly 100 percent of the probiotic you just took. Very little, if any, active probiotic makes it to your colon to recolonize. That said, in certain diseases, there is data to support probiotic use. If, for example, you must take an antibiotic for another illness and you want to prevent the diarrhea associated with that antibiotic, probiotics may help. If you have been diagnosed with irritable bowel disease, probiotics seem to minimally alleviate symptoms. And probiotics can help treat side effects of therapy for *Heliobacter pylori*, the ulcer-causing bacteria.

Should you need probiotics, seek out products containing multiple strains of bacteria. The clinically proven most-active strains are *Saccharomyces boulardii*, *Lactobacillus acidophilus*, *L. casei*, and *L. rhamnosus*. If you have a specific gastrointestinal condition, such as colitis, *H. pylori*, or infectious diarrhea, check with your doctor about what probiotics he or she recommends.

These foods should be a part of your everyday diet. Fiber supercharges your GI tract by bulking up the stool so that it travels through your intestines faster and more frequently. Fiber also helps keep your weight under control, as it adds very few calories to your diet but makes you feel full.

Consider psyllium capsules. Unless you have nutritional restrictions and are under the care of a gastroenterologist, you should be upping your fiber in addition to eating as many leafy vegetables as you can. Keep it simple so you stick with the plan. Take eight fiber capsules, or two tablespoons, of quality fiber like psyllium (without sweeteners) a day. Warehouse clubs like Costco are great sources for high-quality, low-cost fiber.

Avoid fiber biscuits. Yes, you get your fiber, but you also get sugar.

Cast a wary eye on GI supplements. Most supplements that promise to boost your gut health are just another money grab with zero science behind it. Magnesium, for instance, is touted as a hot new nutrient for improving bowel movements—and it does just that. But it's not "new" at all. Milk of magnesia (magnesium hydroxide) and magnesium citrate formulas have been around for decades, if not a century. And they still work, by increasing the speed with which the intestines squeeze stuff through the gut. There are no modern medical studies investigating magnesium supplements for GI health. If you eat green leafy vegetables, whole grains, and tree nuts as I recommend in chapter 3 (see page 223), you will get plenty of magnesium without buying a supplement.

Get a handle on stress. When you experience stress, your sympathetic nervous system kicks in and pulls blood away from your digestive organs into your muscles so you can run away from the stress (the classic fight-or-flight syndrome). Any digestion you were doing stops, and you rapidly have to clear out your colon.

Chapter Cheat Sheet

☐ Find yourself a great primary-care physician—someone you plan on seeing for years to come.

☐ Stay up to date on your vaccinations (and your family's).

☐ Men's health is heart health. Know your blood pressure, know your heart rate, know your cholesterol levels, and take action to keep them where they need to be.

☐ Keep it simple by boosting your immune system with good nutrition, exercise, and sleep. Be sparing in taking supplements—stick with science, not hype, when choosing the right ones.

☐ Avoid antibiotics unless you *absolutely* need them, and a doctor prescribes them.

☐ If you're bleeding from any orifice, go see a doctor.

02

MANATOMY

A Man's Guide to His Body

If only men paid as much attention to their own bodies as they do to what's under the hood of a '68 Ford Mustang GT . . . because what's *under the hood* in the male anatomy is equally fascinating and complex. Whereas many women could draw you a diagram of their reproductive organs, men may feel that their own reproductive function is so simple and there's not much to understand. But you'd be surprised at how many things need to go right in a man's body to make a baby, or maintain healthy erections well into old age, or just to have great sex. And more and more men are realizing that knowing how everything works is the best way to know when something is *not* working the way it's supposed to—and when it might be time to have their testosterone levels checked or book a prostate exam. Men are realizing that when things are working the way they are supposed to, they enjoy a better sex life, more vitality, and a greatly reduced risk of deadlier diseases.

Testosterone: The Molecule, the Myth, the Legend

How is there so much hype around such a small molecule? Many of us equate this hormone with masculinity, and the word is thrown around often to describe anything overtly macho. Unfortunately, all this has obscured the hormone's true significance in men's health. Testosterone has gone through many ups and downs in popularity and is currently a widely prescribed medication for men with low testosterone, a condition called hypogonadism. There's a lot of good about testosterone and testosterone therapy, a little bad, and a lot of hype. As men age, testosterone levels decline. Some physicians and even the FDA argue that decreasing testosterone is a natural sign of aging and, therefore, treating low testosterone associated with aging isn't necessary. I argue, as I wear my reading glasses, that needing glasses is also a natural sign of aging, but I'd hate to stop reading just because I can't see close up as well as I used to. Why would I want to give up the benefits of testosterone therapy just because I'm getting older? It makes no sense. Arthritis and degenerative joint disease are also signs of getting older, but we don't decline knee replacement surgery to our elderly population. Here's all you need to make up your own mind.

THE "T" FACTORY

Testosterone is perhaps the most defining ingredient in a man's body: testosterone, or "T," as the cognoscenti like to call it, is the key hormone for normal male development. Your testicle (testis) makes testosterone when it receives a hormone signal from the pituitary gland, which gets a signal from the brain. Testosterone was part of your development before you were even born. Your mom made testosterone for you while you were developing in

How It Works: Testosterone Production

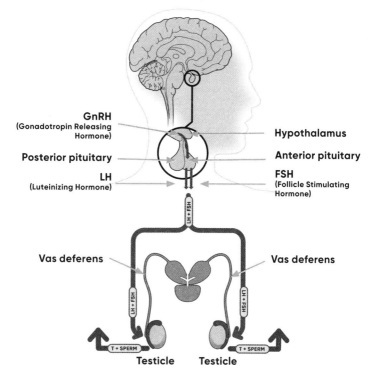

Your brain produces a hormone called GnRH, which stimulates the pituitary gland just below the brain to produce two more hormones, LH and FSH. LH stimulates the testicle to produce testosterone, and FSH stimulates the testicle to produce sperm. The sperm and testosterone then send signals through the bloodstream back to the brain to keep the whole system balanced.

her uterus, and you got just enough of a testosterone boost to trigger your testicles (testes) to drop from your abdomen into your scrotum and to ensure your penis developed properly. Testosterone signals then go dark until puberty. But when puberty hits, T rages back to life, as the gland wakes up the testes and causes you to get erections in algebra class for no reason. When testosterone levels skyrocket, you start making sperm, which you usually continue producing for the rest of your life. Whereas women stop making female hormones after menopause, men produce testosterone their entire life. That said, men will notice declines in testosterone levels and develop low testosterone symptoms the older they get. Each decade a man lives, his chances of developing low testosterone increase by 10 percent or so (a 50-year-old man has a 50 percent chance of hypogonadism). That said, I've seen 80-year-old guys in my practice rocking a 25-year-old's T levels.

WHAT EXACTLY CAUSES LOW T?

It is important for your physician to determine whether your hypogonadism (see page 39) is genetic or acquired. So, as a doctor, if I find your testosterone levels are low, how do I know if I should prescribe medication or meditation? I don't, which is why I like to prescribe both. Decreasing stress through meditation is a great natural T booster. At the same time, if you have an actual hormone deficiency (whether caused by stress or something else), medically treating your deficiency will reduce stress. Sleep is another huge factor in maintaining testosterone levels. When you sleep fewer than six hours a night, your pituitary gland craps out and fails to signal the testicle to make a fresh batch of testosterone overnight. It takes only a night or two of poor sleep to wipe out your T levels.

▶ A CALL TO ACTION Remember when you were 17 and woke up every morning with an erection, could eat anything you wanted and not gain weight? Remember how revved up your libido was? Remember how you could exercise for hours and not get tired? If you're not feeling that level of horniness, energy, or metabolic regulation anymore, consider getting your testosterone checked. Sure, these are all vague symptoms, but they are all associated with low testosterone, so a quick blood test is a good place to start.

KEEPING YOUR T LEVELS TOPPED UP

While a lot of low T is down to genetics, men have more control over their testosterone levels than they think, and much of it has to do with how you live your life. I believe men should first take control of their lifestyle—eating, moving, and sleeping right to boost testosterone.

- Men who stay lean, avoid processed food, and consume a lot of plants, plant proteins, and lean meats tend to have better T levels

- Men who exercise daily have higher T levels

- The best testosterone booster of all? A good night's sleep

Things Your Doctor Can Do to Boost Your T

If your levels are low—under 300 nanograms per deciliter—and your doctor cannot identify an obvious cause, you should seriously consider getting testosterone replacement therapy (TRT). TRT is technically a drug, even if it is a natural hormone. Because TRT is a natural hormone, testosterone therapy has a pretty low risk level. The two big things that will happen as a result of TRT are your red blood cell count will increase, especially if your doctor prescribes injections, and your sperm counts will decrease. (If you are actively trying to conceive, you can't take testosterone unless you are under the care of a male reproductive specialist; see below.) Personally, I love the idea of putting men on short courses of testosterone, just while they are putting their lives back together (it's a myth that once you start T, you're on it forever). There are plenty of ways to recover natural testosterone function after therapy; you just need to find yourself a good endocrinologist or endocrine-trained urologist to guide you. I like to let my patients choose. Many practices, especially stand-alone men's clinics, will force you into whatever that practice is selling, and you'll probably pay a lot more money than going through a traditional physician's office. At my practice, we treat thousands of men with low testosterone, and the treatment methods are pretty evenly divided among the following:

Pills. Testosterone pills have been sold for years. They had a bad record of causing liver damage until a better, newer-generation FDA-approved oral medication called testosterone undecanoate (sold as Jatenzo) became available in 2019. It's taken twice a day with a small meal containing a little fat to help absorption. Men on the new pill will achieve normal testosterone levels with minimal side effects.

Potions. Gel therapy is a safe, effective testosterone delivery system. It's as easy as wiping a teaspoon or so of the gel, which looks and feels like hand sanitizer, onto your shoulders and upper arm every day in the morning. The gel stays active until it dries, so you have to be careful the gel doesn't rub onto anyone else. If your partner or children touch your skin where you applied the gel, they could absorb active testosterone.

Pokes. Injection therapy has been around for decades. When done well, it is a fantastic method. I teach my patients how to inject at home, and they have tightly controlled dosing regimens to keep them at healthy levels.

Procedures. Your physician can insert pellets through a tiny, numbed-up incision into the soft tissue of your backside. The pellets are convenient and offer a steady testosterone level for about four months.

TRT and Fertility

In my practice, some men on testosterone replacement remain fertile, but they are on a complex hormone regimen to specifically preserve fertility. I see too many men and their partners who come to me angry and devastated after some unwise physician prescribed the man testosterone to make him more fertile. Turns out, testosterone therapy is almost a 100 percent effective form of male birth control.

IVAN, 45

What Low T Looks and Feels Like

Ivan is a 45-year-old funds manager. His husband, Paul, is a video-game editor who works from home, and they have 3-year-old twins. They're a busy family, and Ivan is worn out. His libido is much lower than Paul's, and he feels way more stressed than Paul. Ivan has gained about 30 pounds since becoming a father and admits he doesn't exercise much. He can't remember the last time he woke up with an erection, and he avoids intimacy with Paul more than he seeks it. He and Paul used their sperm and a surrogate and egg donor for their twins, and they do not want any more children at this point. Ivan just wants to feel better. He wants more energy, more sex drive, more enthusiasm to work out again.

Ivan had a normal physical exam, and all his general health parameters from vital signs to cholesterol levels checked out well. His testosterone level, however, was 220 nanograms per deciliter—well below the normal value of 300. I spoke with Ivan about testosterone replacement, and he was all in. With his young twins around, I didn't like the idea of his putting a gel on his arms every day, and he admitted he would probably forget to do it most mornings. He had no problem learning to give himself injections. After three months on therapy, Ivan has lost 10 pounds, wakes up most mornings with erections, and he and Paul are delighted with his restored sex drive and desire for intimacy. I see 10 to 15 Ivans a week in my practice because low testosterone is so common and often not diagnosed by primary physicians.

It's shocking how much misinformation there is out there about testosterone replacement therapy—and I've heard it all in my practice. *Will my penis shrink? Does it cause cancer?* Although the answer to most of these questions is no, there are some nuances. Here's a breakdown of everything you're probably wondering.

Myth 1: TRT Will Shrink My Penis

Testosterone therapy will not shrink your penis. I just heard this myth on a popular radio show, so the untruth still gets airplay. Your penis stops being sensitive to testosterone levels once you finish puberty. Some men also think testosterone therapy will enlarge their penises. Believe me, I have taken care of guys who have slathered testosterone gel on their penis hoping it would get bigger, but alas, no effect. *Your testicles, however, will shrink.* Testosterone therapy stops sperm production temporarily; therefore, the testicles contract a bit because there are no sperm to keep them plump. Some guys barely notice. If a man is concerned with loss of testicular size, I can help preserve his size by appropriately dosing him or even adding another hormone medication.

Myth 2: TRT Causes Prostate Cancer

Some doctors still believe this. I'm a fan of science, and science says otherwise. The myth goes back to the Nobel Prize–winning discovery in 1966 that showed that if a man with prostate cancer has his testosterone lowered (surgical or chemical castration), his cancer regresses. For decades, everyone just assumed that if you give a healthy man testosterone, you'll *give* him prostate cancer or make existing prostate cancer worse. Excellent studies now refute this notion, and most urologists and endocrinologists believe that TRT does not cause prostate cancer.

Myth 3: TRT Causes Heart Attack, Stroke, and Blood Clots

Not true, according to all recent randomized, placebo-controlled clinical trials. That said, every man should know his cardiovascular health and risk factors—blood pressure, cholesterol levels, smoking status, family history of heart disease—before beginning any medical treatment or therapy.

SARMs: Designer Testosterone or Overhyped Supplement?

There are things called selective androgen receptor modulators (SARMs) that are all the rage right now—discussed in men's health blogs, podcasts, and random forums. Sounds like something from a sci-fi movie, right? But the science is superinteresting. SARMs, usually in pill form, help the androgen/testosterone molecule bind to specific cells—a muscle cell, a penis cell, a brain cell, and so on—which is a good thing, because testosterone can have a negative effect on some cells if you take too much. SARMs were first studied as a treatment for men with advanced prostate cancer, who have to go on medicine that chemically castrates them. While that keeps the cancer in check, it wreaks havoc on a man's muscle mass, bone density, sex drive, and cardiovascular health. SARMs allowed doctors to give a man a drug that only blocks testosterone in the prostate. The cancer stops growing, but the recipient would have no horrible side effects. Problem is, SARMs didn't work and didn't receive FDA approval. But that didn't stop a whole internet industry from selling SARMs to men. Stay tuned because some day, we may have SARMs that fulfill the promise of designer testosterone therapy, but for now, stay away.

TRT AND RED BLOOD CELLS

TRT can elevate your blood counts. The increase in red blood cell count is rarely dangerous, but your doctor needs to monitor your levels closely and provide recommendations if the levels get too high. Sometimes, men need to give blood (phlebotomy) to normalize their red cell count.

The Penis: An Owner's Manual

Oh, the penis—so much misinformation, so little time to dispel it all. But I will try to cover the most important stuff. Alongside our testes, the penis bears the incredible responsibility of furthering the species. Penises are also truly amazing structures: a lot of physiology goes into this essential part of procreation. The penis has to grow exponentially, and at warp speed, to have the opportunity to ejaculate and procreate. While most "hunting" trips are recreational, not procreational, the mechanics are the same either way because the penis can't tell the difference.

A WORD ABOUT SIZE AND STIFFNESS

This is by far the number one penis question my patients ask me: "Doc, isn't there something you can do to increase my penis size?" The simple and bad news is, no. But you're probably not as small as you think.

Size

Thanks in large part to porn, most men grossly overestimate what normal is when it comes to penis size and the stiffness of their erections. The truth is, the average erect penis is 4.5 to 5.5 inches, and *most* men fall in that range. (Interestingly, for heterosexual couples, that's just right, considering the average vaginal canal is 4 to 5 inches.) When you also take into account that only 20 percent of women orgasm through vaginal penetration, penile size is often less of a factor in great sex than heterosexual men think it is. For the other 80 percent, you just have to be more creative and use more body parts (or toys) to bring a female partner to orgasm. That's a good problem to have. In gay men, size is still an issue less for sexual pleasure but, as for all men, because penile size corresponds to a feeling of adequate manhood. It's an unhappy truth of the male condition.

Erections

A lot of men are surprised when I tell them their penises don't get 100 percent hard when they *feel* as if they have a rock-hard erection. The glans, or tip of the penis, does not get hard. This is by design. The normal blood flow to keep a hard erection is to always have a small amount of spent (deoxygenated) blood leak out of the hard shaft into the glans to shuttle it back to the heart for fresh blood. It is a cycle that lasts as long as the erection. If the glans were rigid as well, the penis would not refill with oxygenated blood. And that would lead to a urologic emergency called priapism which leads to penis damage and erectile dysfunction.

PENIS ENLARGEMENT: THE BIG LIE

One of the most frequently asked questions in my practice is this: *If women can get breast enhancement for small breasts, why can't dudes get penis enhancement for small penises?* Because breast implants expand skin that is pretty elastic and expandable. The penis is an organ with a fixed length and girth. If you stuffed a size enhancer in there, your original penis would be buried. In other words, appreciate what you were born with and heed the following simple advice:

Never Go Under the Knife

Although there are surgical procedures, they are on the fringe of acceptable medical practice, and they often have horrific consequences. Penile enhancement surgeons inject fillers like fat, collagen, and Lord knows what else into a man's penis, or even lacerate the ligaments that keep the penis scaffolded to the pubic bone just to give it a longer dangle (I have operated on too many men for ugly complications of this procedure). Even when the surgery goes right, it does nothing to enhance length! It just gives guys a penis that looks longer when flaccid—a locker-room penis, I call it—and it is actually less functional because the penis has ligaments to keep it anchored during penetration. Guys that get suspensory ligament release end up with an unstable penis and are therefore less functional sexually. Someday, there may in fact be a safe, functional way to improve a man's penis size; until then be wary.

Stay Away from Supplements

Supplements that claim to supersize your penis don't work. Most of them have ingredients like L-arginine, L-citrulline, or even Viagra (adding Viagra is illegal and potentially harmful in over-the-counter supplements). All these do is simply increase blood flow, giving your flaccid penis a little more "show." But as soon as you get an erection, it's the *exact* same erect size as if you never took the supplement.

No, You Can't Stretch It

There is an ancient Middle Eastern technique called jelqing that involves forcibly stretching the penis in hopes of increasing length and girth. Whereas it was once quite fringe, thanks to the internet, jelqing has seen a resurgence. The technique involves initiating a tension response at the base of the penis and milking the tissue toward the head. Most of the time, this is useless and harmless, and I don't dissuade guys from doing it. But some men overdo the jelq and end up hurting themselves. Just remember: no matter how badly you may want a bigger penis, there is no way to safely achieve that goal. Bummer but true.

A Safer Way to Increase Size

One less invasive—some might even say fun—way of increasing size is a cock ring. Cock rings, made of metal, plastic, rubber, rope, silicone, or whatever material is handy, wrap around the base of the penis, or base of the penis and back of the scrotum, to keep the penis more engorged and, thus, slightly larger. Believe it or not, cock rings are medical devices! But then there are sex toy cock rings, jury-rigged cock rings (I've seen industrial steel bolts used), and other creative ways to achieve maximal penile engorgement. If you keep the band or ring on for a short time (well under an hour), then it can help maximize engorgement of the penis during intercourse. But stick with a ring that has a release on it or can easily slide off. If you leave the cock ring on too long, the penis can really swell and make the ring tough to remove. Then the penis starts to die, which is bad. I've had to remove steel rings from penises in the middle of the night with industrial saws—talk about needing a steady hand.

THE CIRCUMCISION DEBATE

More than ever, the foreskin is at the forefront of the zeitgeist. It's no surprise considering there are health, social, *and* religious factors at play when it comes to deciding whether to subject a baby boy to the cut. Let's clear one thing up right off the bat: to date, no professional medical society recommends routine circumcision. If a man does not get circumcised at birth, in all likelihood he'll be fine—we were born that way, after all, and we lived that way for thousands of years before circumcision became a religious and health issue. There is in fact a movement now to not circumcise boys routinely, as advocates think it hurts penile sensitivity, though the scientific literature is pretty sparse on this. Some men are so distraught they were circumcised at birth that they undergo foreskin restoration surgery.

Strictly from a health perspective, circumcision does inhibit HIV transmission in at-risk populations, and it decreases infection rates in men with diabetes (controlling blood sugars is critical to preserving foreskin health). The human papilloma virus (HPV) causes penile cancer, but only in uncircumcised men. Note, however, that an HPV vaccine now exists, and if a boy is vaccinated prior to sexual activity, he's probably not going to get penile cancer.

With all that said, I have no official position on circumcision. It is a personal choice that parents need to make. If you still have your foreskin and it's stretchy, slidey, and doesn't cause you discomfort, it probably is just fine. In fact, many men report that having their foreskin is a big bonus. If, however, your foreskin gets tight, hurts, bleeds, or smells bad, you need to see a urologist. Given higher rates of penile cancer in uncircumcised men, these guys need to pull back that hood daily to make sure there are no spots or lumps and wash the head. Certainly, if a man develops any complications from his foreskin, I would strongly consider circumcision.

The following are a few things to look out for if you still have your foreskin. (If you are circumcised, skip ahead to Peyronie's Disease, Explained.)

Phimosis. This occurs when the foreskin is so tight a man can't pull it back, which can lead to penile infections, an increased risk of sexually transmitted disease, and, rarely, an increased risk of cancer.

The fix: Excellent penile hygiene and gentle retraction on the foreskin, a little bit every day, can improve mild phimosis to the point where a man can fully retract his foreskin. **If you're a parent of an uncircumcised boy, you need to teach him to do this every day once he reaches about six years old.** Steroid creams can improve foreskin retraction, and I usually start with this before I circumcise a man. But the ultimate treatment for phimosis is circumcision. It's an outpatient procedure that takes about a month for full recovery.

Paraphimosis. This is more serious than phimosis. Paraphimosis occurs when the foreskin gets trapped behind the head of the penis and can choke off blood supply to the tip of the penis. This is an emergency.

The fix: Grab the penis tightly and squeeze it hard to help reduce the swelling until you can pull the foreskin back over the head. Then see a urologist immediately, who can figure out why this happened to your penis and reduce the swelling to save the head of the penis from losing blood supply. Ultimately, circumcision is the best treatment here, too.

Frenulum breve. This is when a man's tethering attachment from the head of the penis to the shaft is so short that he can't pull back his foreskin at all and will often tear this skin during sex, which definitely ruins the moment. Most guys want this fixed.

The fix: Frenulum breve has no home remedy. The surgical solution, known as frenuloplasty, is where the urologist cuts the tight band of tissue so the foreskin can slide freely over the head of the penis. Once again, circumcision is also a good answer.

PEYRONIE'S DISEASE, EXPLAINED

Is this the first time you've heard the term Peyronie's disease? I'm not surprised. Many physicians barely know what this devastating condition is. Peyronie's disease is scarring of the penis that leads to penile curving, shortening, and weakening of the erect penis—imagine seeing your penis turn from a straight cucumber to a curvy banana.

Now that there is an FDA approved drug for PD, disease state awareness has increased. If you don't have a curve in your erect penis, consider yourself fortunate—although men can develop PD at any time throughout their adult lives. If you do, know you're not alone.

PD afflicts 10 percent of men. This doesn't seem like a lot of men but the impact Peyronie's has on men and their partners is huge. If you don't have Peyronie's, empathize with guys that do. It can be so bad that men can't engage in penetrative intercourse. Men with Peyronie's also lose substantial length. PD begins as an inflammation in the lining of the penis. The inflammation eventually causes a rigid form of collagen to develop, either overnight or over several months. Once that scar invades the normal penile tissue, chaos ensues—the erect penis bends, anywhere from a gradual curve to greater than 90 degrees! Penetrative sex can become painful, difficult, or even impossible, which can also be psychologically devastating (unsurprisingly, around 40 percent of men with PD suffer from depression). Peyronie's has a strong genetic component, especially in men of Northern European ancestry—I have a Swedish

MIKE, 55

Modern Medicine Saves a Sex Life

Mike developed Peyronie's rather suddenly and had been suffering with a penis that was curved about 60 degrees to the left for five years. He had given up hope on having intercourse with his wife again. He became depressed and avoided intimacy altogether with his wife, and they began a sexless marriage. He came to me to see if there was anything I could do to restore more normal function. I diagnosed him with Peyronie's disease and thought he would be a good candidate for CCH therapy since his strength of erection was good. We began the injections, but he didn't see much improvement after two months of therapy. I also suggested he and his wife meet with a sex therapist to discuss other ways to be intimate without penetrative intercourse. At the last treatment of eight injections over four months, Mike came into my office with his wife. They shared with me that over the last four weeks, they were able to have penetrative intercourse for the first time in over five years. His penis was still curved—he felt about 30 degrees—but even that 50 percent improvement in curvature allowed him to have penetrative sex again. Along with good sex therapy, CCH injections restored this couple's intimacy.

colleague who calls it the Viking disease—and it is not preventable, which is why all the theories about what causes it can be frustrating. Many physicians will tell you Peyronie's happens with rough sex and repetitive trauma to the penis. There is *no* evidence for this. Archaic medical texts blamed Peyronie's on gonorrhea (again, with no evidence).

Treating Peyronie's Disease

Thankfully, treatments for Peyronie's disease are far more proven than the causes. As with most ailments, there are pills, pokes, and procedures.

Pills. While there are no FDA-approved oral medications for PD, many physicians prescribe off-label drugs (an off-label drug is a drug approved by the FDA for other uses that doctors repurpose for a new illness). Pentoxifylline, a drug used to treat lower extremity circulation problems, shows a minimal response rate, with few side effects; most Peyronie's experts—urologists trained in sexual medicine—go to this drug first despite its low efficacy simply because it likely won't make things worse. Colchicine is a gout drug that can reduce inflammation, though you have to take it every day for years for it to have much of an effect. Erectile dysfunction (ED) drugs like sildenafil (Viagra) and tadalafil (Cialis) show minimal efficacy treating Peyronie's.

Pokes. The most exciting treatment in the last few hundred years for Peyronie's is an injection called collagenase clostridium histolyticum (CCH; trade named Xiaflex), a bacterial enzyme that destroys the abnormal collagen scar. It requires eight separate injections, spread over about four and a half months, and between injections, a man has to "model" his penis, which essentially entails stretching and bending the penis for about 90 seconds each day. But CCH will decrease the curvature in a man's penis by about 35 percent, and in some studies more. I've had men that have improved *100 percent*. Now, CCH does have a few scary side effects—bruising, even hematomas or corporal rupture, where the penis literally breaks with an erection—so it is very important you find a urologist who is trained and certified by the FDA to inject this medicine.

Procedures. For men who don't want to wait several months to see results, there are essentially three different types of surgeries for Peyronie's—penile plication, plaque excision and graft, and penile implants (covered in great detail on page 175). But you don't get to choose which you're a candidate for—your penis decides. What I mean is the simpler procedure only works for men with mild curvature, and the complicated procedures are reserved for men with severe deformity.

It's All in Your Head

A surprisingly high number of men experience one of the following odd psychosomatic conditions, which can be tricky to diagnose.

The Guilty Penis

A faithful married man walks into my practice complaining of a reddish, warm, somewhat painful sensation on his penis. He also confesses to a guy's night out in which he visited a strip club and got a lap dance that he never told his partner about. The dance was X-rated, for sure, but he insists there was *zero* skin-to-skin contact. It's what I call guilty penis syndrome—and it's all in his head. Never underestimate the physical manifestation of stress and guilt. The pain and physical sensations are actually completely real, but harmless. I certainly don't advocate adultery— even the soft-core variety—but I do like to reassure men that the burning feeling in their guilty penises is in their big head, not their small one.

The Worried Penis

A close cousin of guilty penis is worried penis, which belongs to a single guy with no attachments who had a night of wild sex with a total stranger and who develops a rash, itch, or burn when he pees. He gets all the proper testing—which would be compulsory in a situation like this—but the tests all come back negative. Basically, he is fixating and feels physical manifestations of his psychological regret. I tell these guys that their penis is built for action and friction and can recover from *most* sexual encounters without long-term consequences.

Testicles: Compact but Mighty

A pair of testicles weighs on average less than two ounces. And yet they perform two of the most critical functions in a man's body: sperm and testosterone production. Since sperm is 50 percent of the human genome, testicles are fighting way above their weight!

WHAT'S IN THE SAC?

Your sac, or scrotum, holds the testicles, and most guys keep this sac tucked warm and tidily away in boxers or briefs. Starting at the top of your scrotum, that bulky stuff up high is your spermatic cord. The cord, about as thick as your pinky, should be pretty soft with even consistency. It contains the sperm tube (aka the vas deferens) and the blood vessels that transport blood to and from the testicle. The cord leads down to the testicle, then veers

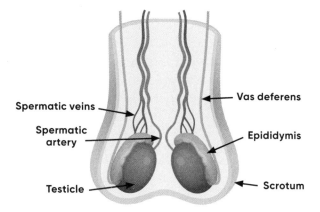

Spermatic veins

Spermatic artery

Testicle

Vas deferens

Epididymis

Scrotum

back up to cradle the testicle, like a spoon cupping an egg. The tender organ that sits on top of the testicle is called the epididymis, and it stores sperm and initiates the ejaculation process. Now on to the testicle itself.

HAPPY, HEALTHY TESTES

The testicles are always fighting to keep cool, as sperm thrives when it is colder than the rest of the body. This is why the scrotum has so many sweat glands: they serve as testicular air-conditioning. Yes, the scrotum may sweat a little more than we want, but it's just trying to keep the testicles cold. (You could go commando from time to time to air out the package.) Meanwhile, all that sweat can cause groin rashes. You might find what look like big pimples on the scrotum. These are sebaceous cysts that, while harmless, can get painful, infected, and large. Don't pop these at home; see your physician, who can numb them and lance them with a sterile technique. Meanwhile, what we call jock itch is usually a fungus. If you notice a red raised patch of skin in your crotch, pick up some over-the-counter Lotrimin cream and apply as the label directs. If that doesn't take care of it in a week or so, make an appointment to see your primary physician. I'm not a fan of drying powders down there—they're messy, and I don't want you breathing in all the dust.

The Self-Exam

Every guy should administer a self-exam on the testicles once a month to make sure everything feels normal. (Testicular cancer can strike us at any age—but it's more common from ages 20 to 60.) Although current preventive medicine guidelines recommend against routine self-exam because most men don't know what they're feeling for (and thus make a lot of unnecessary doctor visits for what is actually normal anatomy), if you follow my easy instructions, you'll get a sense if something isn't right down there and be more informed if you have to go in for a checkup.

Here's what you do:

- Stand in a warm room (so your scrotum is relaxed) or in the shower.

- Gently cup a testicle in your fingertips. Slowly and firmly—but gently—squeeze the testicle from top to bottom and side to side. It should feel smooth and about as squishy as the soft tip of your nose (put one hand on the testicle and one on your nose, if you have to).

- If you feel a harder spot, like the bony part of your nose, in a testicle, see your doctor right away to evaluate for testicular cancer. Testis cancer is rarely painful when it first pops up, but as the tumor grows, it can start to hurt. Testicular cancer is one of the most common cancers in men under age 40, and it spreads rapidly, sometimes doubling in size every day. But it is highly curable if caught early.

TESTICLE TROUBLESHOOTING

Pain of any kind *can* be an indication something is wrong. It may be time to worry if the pain persists for more than an hour, or if certain activities, like vigorous exercise, make it worse. Here is a rundown of the most common things to keep an eye on.

Simple Aches and Inflammation Explained

Most ailments and aches involving your testicles are not that serious: an unlucky shot to the crotch, for example. And sometimes our balls just hurt. There's a lot going on in the scrotum, and all sorts of nerves. Testicles are also extremely sensitive organs, and occasionally you may experience an unexplained twinge of pain.

Simple inflammation *not* caused by infection can be treated with ice and ibuprofen. I see this in men who have recently changed their urinary habits—for example, someone who just returned from a long road trip or flight and didn't get up to pee often enough during his travels.

Vasitis

The vas is the sperm duct that transports sperm from the testicle to the urethra. Some men experience a discomfort called vasitis. To diagnose, squeeze the spermatic cord—the stuff above your testicle—and feel for a thin rope structure (the vas deferens). It normally doesn't hurt to touch; if yours does, you have vasitis. Not much to worry about—simply take some ibuprofen. If you are healthy and don't have heart or kidney disease, you can take

600 milligrams of ibuprofen every 6 to 8 hours for a week to clear up vasitis. That dose is above what the label recommends, so check with your physician to make sure that's okay.

Swollen Veins

When the veins in the scrotum become swollen—which can happen when they are not able to transport blood northward, toward the heart, as they are supposed to—it can create varicose veins in your scrotum, medically termed *varicoceles*. To you, it's an uncomfortable pressure in the scrotum and testicles that often worsens as the day goes on. Varicoceles are actually quite common—15 percent of men have varicoceles, and most men have no symptoms from these big veins. However, varicoceles can impair your fertility and potentially lower your testosterone. Imagine stuffing your scrotum full of gummy worms—that's kind of like what a varicocele feels like. See a urologist so he or she can evaluate your fertility and hormone status. I'll talk more about varicoceles in the fertility section (see page 192).

Epididymitis

This is an infection or severe inflammation in the epididymis, which is the duct that stores and transports sperm. An infection—either a sexually transmitted disease (STD) like gonorrhea or chlamydia, or an infection that originates in the urinary tract—travels up the urethra and down into the epididymis. This can cause a fever, swelling, and even redness over the scrotum. Antibiotics are the answer.

You Feel Severe Pain In One of Your Testicles

This is when the testicle twists and chokes off blood supply. This happens randomly; you can't induce or prevent a torsion. How do you know if you have torsion? If you feel severe pain in one of your testicles—the kind of pain that makes you puke—and it radiates up into your belly, it's time to go to the emergency room. You have about four hours to get into the operating room to save your testicle. Thankfully, the procedure—an orchidopexy—is relatively minor and usually works. Whenever I perform this procedure, I always fix the other testicle, too, because if you get one torsion, you could get two.

Blue Balls: Yes, It's a Real Thing!

Just like a sneeze you can't complete, an ejaculation you don't complete frustrates your central nervous system. The parasympathetic nervous system response builds through arousal, during erection, and during intercourse. At the point of ejaculation, the sympathetic nervous system (your fight-or-flight system) kicks in, delivers an ejaculation, and resets the parasympathetic response. But before you try to persuade your partner to avoid incomplete ejaculation at all costs, you should know that this is *not* dangerous. Besides, you can always take matters into your own hands if he, she, or they are unavailable.

In Praise of the Prostate: A Wellspring of Fertility

Your prostate, ensconced deep in the pelvis, is responsible for making semen—the fluid that enriches and carries sperm—and is, therefore, considered a reproductive organ. It is instrumental in helping sperm travel. Needless to say, it's important to understand the prostate and know how to care for it.

PREVENTIVE PLEASURE

It's true, ejaculating frequently does help the prostate by turning over the fluid more often—cleaning the pipes, as I tell my patients. Other things that boost prostate health are vigorous exercise; a diet rich in antioxidants found in plant-based diets, which decreases the risk of inflammation and may prevent prostate cancer; and maintaining a healthy weight, which combats prostate cancer development. Specifically, eating dark leafy greens like spinach and kale and dark-colored fruits like blueberries and pomegranate is associated with reducing your risk of getting cancer.

THE ORNERY OLD PROSTATE

At around 40 years old, your prostate may begin to enlarge, and it can grow for the rest of your life. Since the prostate surrounds the urethra, if it grows large enough, it will pinch off urinary flow, making it harder to empty the bladder and thus keeping you running to the bathroom all night long. Here are different ways for treating prostate and urinary issues.

Pee Better with a Pill

One of the popular over-the-counter supplements is saw palmetto. While many of my patients say it works for them, I'm not sure saw palmetto lives up to the hype. Many clinical trials show it's no better than taking a placebo pill. But if you see results, go for it. Another over-the-counter supplement is quercetin. There are actually a few clinical trials that show this plant extract settles prostate inflammation. Dosages of all supplements vary based on the manufacturer, so follow directions on the bottle.

When should a man start medication for his urinary symptoms? When he is bothered enough to go on medications with some significant side effects. You may have heard the term benign prostatic hyperplasia, or BPH, and I'm going to tell you it's not so benign. Before we had effective therapies treating enlarged prostates, men could get into a lot of trouble. If a man doesn't empty his bladder fully, he has a higher risk of urinary tract infections, kidney damage, and forming stones in the bladder that need surgical extraction. So, your urologist may prescribe you a prostate drug to prevent these serious conditions.

When a tried-and-true medication is needed, however, I prescribe either an alpha-blocker or a 5-alpha reductase inhibitor (a hormone blocker). Alpha blockers are great drugs with long-term data of effectiveness. They simply relax the prostate muscle so the urinary channel, the urethra, opens up more and the flow maximizes. *However*, about 20 percent of men report no fluid when they ejaculate. They still orgasm, but without release of fluid. Some guys don't mind; other guys think they broke a pipe the first time they orgasm on these drugs. The second type of medication, the 5-alpha reductase inhibitor, *shrinks* the prostate by blocking a key hormone the prostate needs. It has very good long-term effects and is overall very safe, although about 10 percent of men will lose their libidos. An even smaller number will get gynecomastia (swollen breast tissue) and nipple sensitivity. Libido loss usually returns when men stop the drug, but this side effect dissuades many men from taking these drugs.

Pee Better with a Procedure

If pills don't work, or if a man hates the side effects, there are procedures like prostate steaming, trademarked as Rezum. Your urologist injects steam into multiple locations in the prostate through a camera-guided tube (a cystoscope) in the urethra. The enlarged prostate tissue melts away, and after a few weeks, the man starts to pee much stronger (though he has to wear a catheter for a couple of days, until the internal swelling goes down). The real benefit to Rezum is it doesn't seem to affect a man's ability to ejaculate (the biggest risk of most surgeries). Another new procedure is called prostate arterial embolization, or PAE, where an interventional radiologist chokes off the blood supply to the obstructing part of the prostate using X-ray-guided plugs. As the blood supply dies, the prostate tissue shrinks and the urinary channel opens up. The advantage to both Rezum and PAE is most men preserve ejaculatory function. The minimally invasive nature of these procedures makes them popular, but they aren't as effective as surgery to improve urination.

Pee Better with Surgery

The granddaddy of prostate surgeries is the suprapubic prostatectomy, where the surgeon makes an incision in the lower abdomen and shells out the prostate. It's a fantastic surgery for big prostates and more effective than less-invasive surgeries. Many surgeons perform this surgery with the assistance of a robot to minimize recovery time and complications. If I had, or ever develop, a huge prostate, this is the way I'd go. Another less-invasive surgery that scrapes out excess prostate tissue is performed via a cystoscope inserted in the urethra up to the prostate. Known as the transurethral prostatectomy (TURP), many call this one the "Roto-Rooter." Again, the biggest risk of any surgery for enlarged prostate is loss of ejaculation. Orgasms are still good, but no fluid will come out with the finish. Since the medications cause this same side effect, most men understand that's the price they pay to pee purposefully.

SOME GOOD NEWS ABOUT PROSTATE CANCER

Prostate cancer is the second most common cancer in men, after skin cancer. Somewhere around one in six guys will develop it, which is about 300,000 American men every year. Black men are more prone to developing it at a younger age than men of other races. More men die from prostate cancer than any other malignancy—but that is only because it is so common. **The important takeaway here is that if caught early, prostate cancer is one of the most curable cancers out there.** Only 10 percent of men diagnosed with prostate cancer will die from it.

▸ **A CALL TO ACTION** ◂ **Your responsibility as a man is to get your blood levels tested for prostate-specific antigen (PSA) somewhere around age 50.** If you have a father or brother who developed prostate cancer before age 60, then you should get checked while you're in your 40s. Most current medical guidelines recommend prostate cancer screening between the ages of 45 and 55, depending on family history.

Know your risk of prostate cancer and get screened! There are few things more tragic in medicine than seeing a man with incurable prostate cancer. If he had known, or someone who loved him knew, to be checked after he turned 50, he wouldn't have to die from the disease.

The Prostate Exam

Most men are uncomfortable with the thought of having a person's finger in their rectum. The digital rectal exam (DRE) is pretty straightforward; the healthcare provider inserts a lubricated, gloved finger about an inch into the man's rectum, checks the anus and prostate for lumps, and gets an idea of how big the prostate feels. It takes 15 seconds and can save your life. Just get it done—somewhere around age 50, and after talking about the risks and benefits with your healthcare professional.

TREATING—AND BEATING— PROSTATE CANCER

Treatment choices and prognosis depend on a few things: how old the man is, how aggressive the cancer is, and how advanced the cancer is.

Some prostate cancers are so slow growing that men can live the rest of their lives without needing treatment. In those cases, many doctors prefer

MARCUS, 55

Early Detection and a Happy Ending

55-year-old Marcus was healthy, ate well, exercised regularly, and slept a solid seven hours or more every night. But his erections were not as strong as they used to be, and he wasn't waking up with erections. He made an appointment with me to figure out what was going on. During my comprehensive evaluation, I asked if he had been screened for prostate cancer, as he was at that age and, as a Black man, had a higher incidence of developing prostate cancer at a younger age. His dad had had prostate cancer 20 years earlier and beat it with a course of radiation therapy. Marcus didn't see a doctor regularly since he was so healthy. I examined him and didn't find anything concerning, but I recommended he have blood work done to check male hormone levels like testosterone and to measure prostate-specific antigen (PSA) to screen for prostate cancer. I also started him on oral medication to treat his erectile dysfunction. When his blood test came back high, suggesting he had a significant risk of prostate cancer, I recommended he undergo an MRI of his prostate and, potentially, a biopsy. Indeed, the MRI revealed a suspicious area on the prostate, and the subsequent prostate biopsy showed Marcus had early-stage aggressive prostate cancer that was curable. He decided, after much counseling, to have his prostate removed by one of my outstanding urologic oncology colleagues. Using a surgical robot, my colleague removed Marcus's prostate, and Marcus left the hospital the morning after his surgery. He was back in my office in two months and felt great. His erections were starting to return on the therapy I prescribed, and he was grateful we had the discussion about screening for prostate cancer. There are no symptoms of early prostate cancer—Marcus's erectile dysfunction was incidental, but thankfully, that brought him to my office, so I had a chance to check him out thoroughly.

active surveillance of the cancer, which can include following the tumor with blood tests, an MRI, and occasional tissue biopsies, because there are no side effects. In general, men diagnosed in their 70s or 80s probably won't need to be treated aggressively. If you have a less-aggressive cancer that hasn't spread, you have at least 10 years of living before you have to worry that the cancer could cause much harm.

If a man is diagnosed with a moderate to aggressive cancer, and he's under 70 and healthy, there are two mainstream treatments: radiation and surgery.

Radiation Therapy

This is an option for men who do not want surgery or are not healthy enough to undergo surgery. Radiation slowly burns the cancer's blood supply to kill the tumor. Treatment is tolerable but no walk in the park; it can last from 5 to 40 days, depending on the dosing schedule. Mild side effects of radiation include frequency of urination, loose stool, and fatigue. Men will also develop erectile dysfunction, but usually not right away (it can take months to years). Some men experience severe side effects, including blood in the urine, injury to the rectum that can lead to chronic diarrhea, and blood in the stool.

Radical Prostatectomy

This is the surgical removal of the prostate and the seminal vesicles. While the prostate is a vital organ for sexual and reproductive function, it is not essential for life. Nevertheless, this is a big surgery in which the surgeon has to cut out the prostate, sew the urethra and bladder back together, and preserve the erectile nerves that course along the perimeter of the prostate. Erectile dysfunction happens in about 50 percent of men undergoing this surgery.

However, there are newer scientific protocols and therapies that can prevent such high rates of ED that you should ask your surgeon about before going under the knife. At UCLA, men go through "pre-hab." It's a program I developed where we see men before their prostate surgery to counsel them on nutrition and exercise, start them on ED medications ahead of the surgery, and instruct them on using a vacuum erection device. Men who comply with this therapy statistically recover better erectile function.

Chapter Cheat Sheet

☐ If you suspect you are in need of testosterone replacement, learn the facts before you commit, and don't start taking testosterone if you're trying to initiate a pregnancy.

☐ Give your scrotum some respect. It's a complicated sac that includes the testicles—learn the anatomy and what can go wrong.

☐ Your penis is an evolutionary miracle; one pipe that does two jobs, urinate and procreate. Take care of it, respect it, learn to appreciate it for what it is, and be confident that it is most likely the right size.

☐ Your prostate is a sexual organ that makes semen. But it can cause trouble, from urination issues to cancer. Get yours checked regularly once you hit age 50.

☐ For any man with prostate urinary issues, there are lots of treatment options. Learn them so you're informed when you talk with a urologist.

☐ If you are diagnosed with prostate cancer, take action—early detection maximizes chances of cure.

03

EAT

A Man's Guide to Nutrition

Life on earth is sustained by food, water, and sex. Without food and water, we die; without sex, we don't procreate. What you eat and drink fuels great sex and optimal fertility. The key to a healthy man is good nutrition. Meanwhile, nutrition is one of the most confusing subjects to understand. Multiple industries mislead you into buying foods and products they say are healthy but may, in fact, be crap. Mixed messages are everywhere. In this chapter, I hope to explain how to simplify your trips to the grocery store and master a few simple meals. Just a few key tools will go a long way in fueling your body and optimizing your health, your weight, and, yes, your sex life.

Understanding Your "Ideal" Weight

There is no exact scientific definition of "ideal" weight. You can weigh 150 pounds and be over-weight *or* underweight—it depends on how tall you are, but it also depends on how much fat you're carrying. Being overweight is obviously unhealthy. But if you're too skinny, that's not healthy either. Figuring your own "ideal" weight is the first step in achieving your goal.

BMI DOESN'T TELL THE WHOLE STORY

The body mass index (BMI) has long been considered the primary reference point for a person's health. It's even considered a *vital* sign. If you have a high BMI, it simply means you're wider than you should be for your height. But be aware that BMI is nothing more than a ratio, and it doesn't tell the whole health story. Sure, referencing BMI is not a bad way to tell a sedentary guy he's overweight. But if you were to test the BMI of elite-skills athletes in football, even ones with 8 percent body fat, their BMIs would land them in the obese category. A lot of NFL running backs tend to be short, for instance, but they play at about 225 pounds. A six-foot tailback playing at 225 pounds has a BMI of 30.5, which is obese, according to the ratio. Take one look at that athlete's six pack and you know he's not obese. Clearly, BMI is only part of the health equation. It's a reasonable tool if you're the average sedentary guy. But you're not; that's why you're reading this book! If you must know your BMI, see below for how you get that number.

HOW-TO
Calculate BMI

Take your weight in pounds, multiply by 703, and divide by your height in inches squared. That is some complicated math, so you can instead enter your weight and height into any online BMI calculator and get your answer without having to remember exponential division.

Here's a chart of where BMI lines up to ideal weights.

Underweight	BMI less than 18.5
Normal weight	BMI 18.5–24.9
Overweight	BMI 25–29.9
Obese	BMI 30 or higher
Morbidly obese	BMI 35 or higher

WAIST SIZE IS THE THING TO WATCH

Rather than relying on BMIs, I much prefer using a man's waist size to determine his ideal weight. Imagine a 6-foot, 255-pound, out of shape guy compared to the 6-foot, 225-pound running back I mentioned on the previous page. They both have the same BMI, but the sedentary guy has a 40-inch waist and the running back has a 32-inch waist. The 32-inch guy is way healthier and likely has better heart health, because we know that the more weight a guy carries around his beltline, the higher his risk of heart disease. Here's how that applies to you: If you were fit in high school, try to remember your waist size back then and see where you're at now. If you've been hitting the weights, you've probably put on some pounds but more or less maintained that high school waist size. But if you've been hitting the beer and pizza, you've probably let out several notches on your belt. There is no ideal waist size, as bone structure has something to do with it. But it's pretty tough to be in great, heart-healthy shape if your waist measures more than 38. Being 36 or under likely means you're doing okay. If you want to get shredded and slim down to 32, go for it. But you don't need a six pack to be heart healthy and live longer.

A CALL TO ACTION Regardless of what you weigh, too much belly fat kills. You've probably heard this before. Men who carry weight around their midsection have a much higher risk of heart disease. Lower-body fat distribution (that is, around the hips and thighs) tends to be less harmful for men. It turns out that fat is very metabolic and needs a lot of blood flow to maintain itself. Belly fat steals blood away from the heart. When a potbellied man exerts himself, his heart isn't getting as much blood as it needs, and this puts him at risk of a heart attack.

Losing Weight for Life

If you're trying to get back to your high school weight, it's likely a struggle. Yes, there are plenty of trendy diets—meaning temporary changes in your eating habits—that can lead to weight loss. **But from a men's health angle, I'm not a fan of diets. I prefer that you change your *relationship* to food and your weight, and figure out a life plan that works for you**. In fact, I don't think diets work. But I do get that you may need to lose a bunch of weight fast to kick-start the process. The key is understanding which diets work for what and how to transition into a *sustainable* approach to nutrition. Remember, a diet is a quick fix at best, but your relationship with food and health is a lifelong adventure.

DIETS ARE BS—*ALL* DIETS

Please, if you take one message about nutrition from this book, it's that *all diets will fail*. To be clear, I'm talking about those temporary, often unrealistic regimens designed to help you shed pounds fast. The worst diets are the rapid-weight-loss plans that deliver instant results—I'm looking at you, keto, a uniquely instant weight dropper with a horrible bounce back if you fall off the wagon. Even the most popular diets, where people do end up losing a ton of weight, will eventually fail. They suck you into the short-term goal of how you look, but they are not at all sustainable. Unless you are willing to stay on a diet forever, you *will* regain the weight. What's the alternative? Change the way you engage with food; change what food means to you.

A NEW FOOD PHILOSOPHY

The best diet for a man is simply a plan he can stick with. Then it's not a diet—it's a new way of life. Which is why I prefer simple *rules* to any diet: eat lots of veggies, consume a little meat, and take in fewer calories each day. **Ideally, 60 percent of the food on your plate should be veggies with no added oils or sugary sauces, 30 percent should be lean proteins, and 10 percent should be complex carbohydrates (whole-grain pasta or bread, for example).** Be aware, however, that a simple combo of meat, starch, and veggies is not always healthy, as illustrated below.

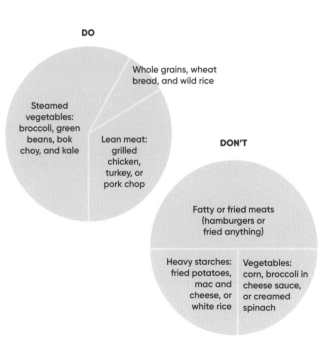

DO

Whole grains, wheat bread, and wild rice

Steamed vegetables: broccoli, green beans, bok choy, and kale

Lean meat: grilled chicken, turkey, or pork chop

DON'T

Fatty or fried meats (hamburgers or fried anything)

Heavy starches: fried potatoes, mac and cheese, or white rice

Vegetables: corn, broccoli in cheese sauce, or creamed spinach

The top plate on the previous page shows a good balance of lean meats, whole grains, and green vegetables.

The bottom plate shows fatty meat and potatoes and vegetables drenched in cheese sauce. Both plates are equal parts meat, starch, and vegetable, but the top plate will give you the nutrition you need, while the bottom plate will give you heartburn and a bigger belly.

 MANUEL, 42

A Man Who Had Had Enough

I've worked with Manuel for years. He's one of my favorite surgical techs. Manny was always a big guy—over 350 pounds. But I hadn't been in his operating room for more than a year, and when I saw him recently, I didn't recognize him because he had lost so much weight: 100-plus pounds! I asked him how he did it, and he said, "Simple, Doc. I stopped eating so much, and I started walking." Manny was done with feeling terrible, falling asleep when he got home, not spending quality time with his kids. And he's kept the weight off. He tells me all the old fatty foods he loved make him sick now. After sticking to his new eating plan, he changed his life forever. Specifically, Manny converted his diet so it features minimal dairy, lots of green vegetables, and allows far less meat consumption. And every day he walked a little farther than the day before. He's dropped enough weight that he's now lifting weights and jogging a little—and he wants to keep going another 20 pounds.

THE CLOSEST THING
TO A SHORTCUT

Listen, if you don't have time to eat perfectly, follow these four simple rules and you will at least eat much better, likely lose weight, and have more energy:

1. **Stop eating fast food**—completely. Fast food is not *real* food. It's not enough to say you'll stick with fast-food salads and avoid the burgers. The salads are loaded with calories, too. Once you're used to a diet full of whole, fresh food, those burgers and fried foods feel like a pound of regret in your belly.

2. **Avoid sugar at all costs, and never add sugar to anything (we'll talk more on how harmful sugar can be on page 95).** In our American diet, sugar seems to find its way into everything, from smoothies to whole-wheat bread to organic yogurt. Sugar—even natural sweeteners like agave, honey, maple syrup, or fruit syrups—is loaded with calories. Eliminate sugar, and your body will adjust within a week or two to the point where you will not like sweet foods anymore.

3. **Stay away from processed foods (see more on the next page).** Cook your own food, using real ingredients that you don't have to unwrap or take out of a box.

4. **Quit all drinks except water, black coffee, or unsweetened tea.** Sodas, energy drinks, and juices are packed with calories. Quaffing three 16-ouncers of your favorite unhealthy beverage is like eating a stick of butter.

A FEW TOOLS FOR IMMEDIATE WEIGHT LOSS

Sometimes, a man does need to lose a lot of weight quickly for health reasons, and this requires a nuanced approach. In these cases, it makes sense to employ a few extreme measures at first, before focusing on lifestyle. Here are some effective short-term tactics:

Count calories. The body is a machine, and food is fuel. If you burn more fuel or take less fuel in, your body will burn fat, which is stored energy.

Choose between low-carb or low-fat. If you like steak, try a low-carb diet. If you like potatoes, know that you'll have to go on an extremely low-fat diet to lose any weight. In general, low-fat diets are the hardest to lose weight on. That's because with carbohydrates, it's so easy to eat a lot of calories before feeling full. High-fat, low-carb diets are easier for shedding pounds because fats are filling.

Avoid processed foods. Not all processed foods are bad, but the fewer ingredients and fewer steps it takes to create a food, the better. Here's a simple way to tell if something is processed or not: if you can't grow it, forage it, or kill it, it's processed. That leaves a big list—bread is processed, cheese is processed, yogurt is processed . . . and so on. It's especially important to avoid packaged food with added sugar, fat, or salt. This weight-loss tactic entails resetting your relationship with food. Know that those greasy, sweet, processed foods you ingest now taste great because you're used to them; you expect you'll experience a little heartburn, feel a bit bloated, gain weight from those foods, and you're okay with that. To lose weight, you have to trust that the new way of eating will become your norm and that you'll lose your appetite for processed foods. It's been more than 10 years since I've set foot in a national burger chain, and I feel sick even thinking about eating that kind of junk again.

Weight-Loss Supplements Warning

There are no supplements that will help you lose weight. Those that say they will are probably dangerous, containing a stimulant that works just like caffeine. You've probably read about chromium, goji berry, garcinia cambogia, and a bunch of others—they don't work. Please, do not waste your money. Supplement manufacturers have no regulatory body, so they can claim *whatever* they want about their products and put anything they want into that little bottle.

CHOOSE A NEW APPROACH TO EATING

Lots of studies have shown effective weight-loss programs from keto to Atkins to extreme low fat (like Dr. Ornish) to intermittent fasting. They all work. But remember, the results are only temporary. Likewise, ketogenic diets do burn fat, preferentially, and are probably safe in the short term. But it is hard to stay compliant long term, and when you fall off the wagon onto a big jelly doughnut, you'll regain the weight. Take a look at how each diet works (and doesn't work) in the following chart and choose an approach that could become a lifestyle.

Pick a Plan

You should individualize your diet for how *you* want to eat. The following chart distills many popular diets into what the rules are, what the science is, and what is good and bad about each one. Remember, I don't believe in diets for a long-term solution to your relationship with food. But I do believe some guys need fast results and therefore there's a role for diets in your health overhaul. So, if you're trying to lose weight fast, read on and pick a plan!

THE DIET	THE DOS	THE DON'TS	THE SCIENCE	PROS	CONS
Low carb (Atkins, South Beach)	Fatty meats Butter Cream cheese Tree nuts Leafy veggies Cauliflower Minimal fruit	Sugar Bread Wheat pasta	Hard to eat a lot because eating calorie-dense food when the body is sugar depleted will burn fat instead	Rapid weight loss Decreases blood sugar—may be good for limiting diabetes risk	Rapid weight gain once off the diet Low fiber Nausea Diarrhea Body odor
Ketogenic ("keto")	Same as low-carb diets, but majority (70 percent) of calories are from fat	Sugar Fruit Bread or grains Wine or beer (hard alcohol okay)	Body goes into ketosis and burns fat (there is no sugar to burn)	Same as low-carb diets Some science that keto is good for controlling epilepsy, may be good for controlling cancer growth	Same as low-carb diets

Intermittent fasting	Eat what you want, but only in a small (8-hour) window	Eat for 16 hours of the day	Significant calorie reduction Body goes into starvation mode Makes it difficult to binge Stomach shrinks	Rapid weight loss No food restrictions No known health problems May increase longevity	Rapid weight gain once off the diet Hunger, especially during early days Hard to exercise on fasting diets until the body fully converts to starvation mode
Low fat (i.e., Ornish diet)	Lots of veggies and fruit Nonfat dairy Whole grains Minimal meats Sugar okay	Butter and oils (including olive oil) Fatty meats like bacon, burgers, sausage Eggs Alcohol Regular cheese Milk	Fats are high in calories Difficult to overeat with vegetables and whole-grain breads, therefore reducing calorie intake If the man stays compliant, extreme low-fat diets are proven to reverse heart disease	Heart healthy Lots of veggies Pretty much eliminates all processed foods	Compliance superhard: humans crave fat! Hard to feel satisfied Can end up eating a lot of sugar

THE DIET	THE DOS	THE DON'TS	THE SCIENCE	PROS	CONS
Paleo	If you can kill it or forage it, you can eat it Meat and veggies	Processed food Dairy Grains Potatoes	Eat like your ancestors Based on hunter-and-gatherer diets No good scientific studies, but diet makes some sense	No processed food Good meat and veggie balance Can eat good balance of fat, protein, and carbs Lots of tree nuts and fish	Hard to meal prep Expensive
Whole 30	For 30 days, eat meat, potato, tree nuts, vegetables, seeds, seafood, fruits, fats (even clarified butter)	Sugar Grain Alcohol Beans Dairy (except clarified butter)	None! It's all made up, with some basis in common sense	Eliminates processed food Lots of veggies and fruit	Compliance difficult No science High fat Expensive Unbalanced

A LAST RESORT FOR WEIGHT LOSS

Surgery is an extreme measure, but it can save your life. For any man who has reached a point where diet and lifestyle changes won't reverse his obesity fast enough, and he simply can't get the weight off any other way, bariatric surgery—procedures like gastric bypass or gastric sleeve—may be an option. To find a qualified bariatric surgeon in your area, go to the American Society for Metabolic and Bariatric Surgery website at asmbs.org and enter your zip code. It's not an easy, quick fix, however, and not one to take lightly. You will still have a lot of work to do with your diet after the procedure. But surgery can shed the pounds and reduce your risk of diabetes, high blood pressure, and a host of other severe illnesses.

The basic principle of bariatric surgery is to shrink your stomach so you feel full before you eat too many calories. Problem is, you can drink thousands of calories before you feel full. Every sugary soda, energy drink, or glass of wine or beer contains 150 to 200 calories. If you have gastric-reducing surgery and don't pay attention to food and drink, you could drink right through any stomach shrinking and eliminate any weight reduction. You must change your mind-set before you can change your body. If you're considering surgery, it's a good idea to stop drinking calories for a month to see how you feel and how much weight you lose *without* the surgery. Then, if you decide to go through with it, you still shouldn't drink your calories afterward.

SEE A DOCTOR IMMEDIATELY IF . . .

You Experience Unexplained Weight Loss

With obesity rates in this country at an all-time high, weight loss is rarely a bad thing. However, if you're not trying to lose weight and you're dropping pounds, you need to get checked out. Sometimes it's an issue with your thyroid gland. Or it could be anything from intestinal parasites to depression or stress to not getting enough sleep. But unexplained weight loss is also a hallmark of cancer. Cancer is metabolically expensive, meaning it needs a lot of calories to grow, and it robs your body of the calories you're taking in. In short, if you're losing a lot of weight without trying, see your primary physician, who can order the appropriate tests and refer you to specialists to treat you.

Shop Smarter, Cook Simpler, Eat Better

Ever hear the expression "Abs are made in the kitchen"? You can do as many ab crunches as you want in the gym, but you'll still have a load of laundry covering your washboard if you don't eat for a fit body. I say, "Abs are made in the grocery store." You have to buy the right ingredients and avoid throwing calorie-bomb foods into your cart so they don't even make it to your cupboard. You can have a refrigerator full of kale and nonfat Greek yogurt, but if you have a can of Pringles or a pint of ice cream, what do you think you'll reach for? I know better than to tempt myself. If I need to cut back on calories, I keep the nutritional sabotage out of my house altogether. Eating to be a healthy man isn't as hard as it seems. And it shouldn't have to cost you half of your paycheck. It does require discipline and a shift in your mind-set, but once you stick to a lifestyle change, you'll never go back to your old ways.

WHOLE FOOD VERSUS PROCESSED FOOD

A whole food is anything not altered or minimally altered. A baked potato with butter or bacon is a whole food. French fries: not a whole food. A baked chicken breast is a whole food. A fried breaded chicken nugget: not a whole food. Brown whole-grain rice is a whole food. White rice: not whole. White rice is stripped of all its nutritional value and reduced to essentially a grain of sugar.

HEALTHY EATING DOES NOT NEED TO BE EXPENSIVE

Packaged or processed food is actually far more expensive than whole foods (especially if you buy in bulk). Eating right does, however, require more time—but you will definitely save money. Here are three great ways to cut costs and eat better:

1. Stop obsessing over organic.

   The USDA Organic certification simply means produce is grown without pesticides and meats come from animals that have not been fed hormones, antibiotics, or pesticide-treated grain. Is organic any more nutritious than nonorganic food? Nope. Sugar, for example, is pretty darn evil, whether it's organic or not. That all said, pesticides are certainly a concern. The truth is, superharmful pesticides have been banned in the United States for decades, and the residual pesticide you ingest from nonorganic produce is minimal. I personally believe that if you can afford it, buy organic—it's better for the planet (reducing groundwater pollution and honeybee/pollinator stress), better for small farmers (reducing their exposure to chemicals), and *maybe* a tiny bit better for you. If you choose organic and have a schedule that permits, farmers' markets are great places to pick up fresh produce. But if you're not eating healthy produce because you can't afford organic, stop worrying. Buy nonorganic food, then wash it really well—just as you should with organic produce. (By the way, illness-causing *E. coli* is 100 percent organic and can infect organic lettuce just as easily as nonorganic lettuce.) Some experts recommend washing your produce in dilute vinegar or baking soda to kill any surface bacteria, but simple running water is good enough. Most organic produce is washed with a dilute chlorine solution (the same chemical used in tap water).

Philosophically, do I want the world to be a better place and revert to simple farming and organic production? Sure, but let's work on you first.

2. Rethink meat portions.

Lean, nutritionally dense meat protein such as chicken or fish is indeed pretty expensive. But we should all be cutting back on our meat protein. I recommend your meat consumption per meal at 4 to 5 ounces. Load your plate with other options—vegetables, whole-grain rice, beans, or ancient grains like quinoa. These will fill you up, provide balanced nutrition, extend that chicken breast or sustainable low-mercury fish so that it lasts a couple of days, thereby halving your meat expense. For an up-to-date list of responsible fish choices, check out seafoodwatch.org. The Monterey Bay Aquarium runs the site and offers healthy recipes with sustainable fish like salmon, char, and trout.

3. Get a couple of kitchen gadgets.

A rice cooker or pressure cooker will expand your menu options and reduce your budget *and* waistline. But you don't need a lot of special equipment to eat well. I once had a kitchen full of pots, pans, food processors, bread makers, espresso machines, and high-end knives. Then my wife and I realized we didn't need 80 percent of what we owned—it just cluttered the kitchen. Now we cook every day and almost never eat out. These are the items we can't live without:

- **High-performance blender** for making smoothies
- **Pressure cooker/multicooker** for quickly cooking beans and whole grains
- **Food processor** for chopping vegetables, making sauces
- **Espresso maker** for preparing morning coffee
- **Steel soup pot** for boiling whole-wheat noodles

Understand Your Macros

A macronutrient is any food molecule that has a caloric value. Proteins, fats, carbohydrates, and alcohols are all macros, and each has a calorie value per gram. When trying to lose or maintain weight, you have to burn more—or at least the same amount—of calories in a day than you eat. Therefore, some simple back-of-the-envelope math can go a long way. A carbohydrate has four calories per gram, protein also has four calories per gram, alcohol has seven calories per gram, and fat has nine calories per gram. Simply put, a gram of fat has more than twice the calories of a carbohydrate.

KNOW A SUPERFOOD FROM A SUPERFAD

Acai, goji, pomegranate, blueberry—go ahead, name your dark fruit of the month. These are just a few of the fruits touted as superfoods. But nothing really makes these fruits that super other than they have a better agent and marketing team. There is no federal superfoods committee that decides who makes the list and who doesn't. Is kale a superfood and spinach not? They have a similar nutrient profile, but kale is so sexy now that many folks think it is better than spinach. The fact is, all dark-green leafy vegetables and dark berries are high in antioxidants and phytochemicals. These properties may help prevent cancer, but they are not unique to the trendy foods that get the press. There is no one superfood. Unfortunately, most companies that tout superfoods as ingredients (in things like acai bowls) are also loading their products with sugar. Look at the nutritional labels and strive to eat foods in their purest form. Instead of buying a premade acai bowl, for instance, prepare your own bowl of whole-grain oatmeal, nonfat Greek yogurt, and acai berries with a sprinkling of coconut flakes on top. That's a super eating plan.

KNOW THY ENEMY: SUGAR

Technically, man can live without eating sugar (as with the keto diet). The question is, can we live well? Eating sugar does release dopamine, our feel-good hormone, because sugar is quick energy that wards off starvation, according to our primitive brain. The problem is, sugar is delicious. Over the last few centuries, it has become so abundant that most of us eat way too much of the sweet stuff. And it makes us fat. You see, once our sugar storage center in the liver is full—which, by the way, doesn't take much—our bodies put the excess into long-term storage: fat cells. For all the effort someone might put into eating the right kinds of sugar, the truth is our bodies don't care one bit how it gets sugar. Brown, turbinado, minimally refined, organic, beet, raw—there is no "healthy" form of sugar. The healthiest sugar is the sugar you don't eat! Never add sugar to anything ever again. Never drink another sugared soda or energy drink. And don't be fooled into thinking some sugars are better than others.

TYPE	SOURCE	CALORIES PER GRAM
White sugar	Sugarcane, sugar beet	4
Brown sugar	Sugarcane	4
Turbinado sugar	Sugarcane	4
Corn syrup	Corn	4
High-fructose corn syrup	Corn, laboratory	4
Honey	Bees	3–4
Maple syrup	Maple tree	3
Agave syrup	Agave cactus	4
Molasses	Sugarcane, sugar beet	3

Skip Cold Pressing

There's a thought that standard pressing destroys the nutrients in the juice, and so you have to go cold pressed. Cold-press juicing does not remove the sugar in the juice, but it removes the fiber, so you're stuck with a lot of sugar, and no fiber to slow down sugar absorption and the resulting insulin release. The argument that cold pressing maintains the nutrient balance doesn't offset the sugar surge and weight-loss sabotage.

An Exception to the Sugar Rule: Whole Fruit

Yes, whole fruit is full of natural sugar. But it also has a ton of fiber, and fiber blunts the effect of sugar on your body. Take an apple, for example: if you eat an apple—peel and all—your body metabolizes the sugar slowly and your sugar levels won't spike to the point where your body starts converting sugar into fat. The fiber in the apple fills you up, and you stop eating. Eat a bowl of applesauce, however, and by losing the peel, that fruit causes your sugar levels to spike a little higher, spurring you to eat more applesauce. Therefore, it takes more sugar to feel full. Drinking apple *juice* is no different than drinking a couple of ounces of pure sugar. In Los Angeles, I can walk into a shop and pay eight bucks for a cold-pressed juice and feel superhealthy and smug about myself. But what I really did was drop eight bucks on a bucket of delicately pressed sugar.

SALT IS ESSENTIAL

For some reason, salt has gained a reputation as being bad for us—or at least a substance that should be a rare indulgence. But we need salt to live. The entire human body, from heart to kidneys to brain, runs on salt. Salt allowed us land dwellers to crawl out of the briny ocean thousands of years ago to roam the earth. So why are we always being told to cut back on our salt intake? Because too much of a good thing is a bad thing, and the typical American diet overshoots recommended salt intake by *double*, if not more. If you eat out often or eat a lot of processed foods, I guarantee you're getting more salt than you need. Your kidneys do a pretty good job of processing the extra sodium, but if you take in too much salt and don't excrete enough (say, by doing sweaty exercise), your kidneys can't keep up, which leads to high blood pressure.

No, you do not need to start weighing your salt. But I do want you to be smart about your salt intake, which comes back to limiting processed food and how often you eat out. And when you cook, don't add any more salt than the recipe calls for. On the other hand, if you're working out hard and sweating a ton, you might actually need a little *extra* salt. Add electrolyte tablets to your water after any sweaty workout that lasts longer than 30 minutes (avoid the toxic premade sports drinks—more on that later).

A quick word on designer salt. Salt is a simple chemical compound, equal parts sodium and chloride, or NaCl. Your body doesn't care if your salt comes from Kansas or Nepal. Himalayan pink salt, black salt, sea salt, iodized salt, salt off the backs of Amazonian tree frogs (pretty sure I made that one up, but I wouldn't be surprised): from a health perspective, these salts all have minerals that contribute to their nuances in taste but don't change their nutritional content in any significant way. Your body needs the sodium and chloride in salt to live and produce electricity to drive cellular function. The extra minerals in fancy salts will drive up the price but not result in a healthier product. In fact, people who live in the Himalayas and eat exclusively Himalayan salt have a very high rate of goiter, a thyroid condition associated with iodine deficiency. (Most table salt in the United States has iodine added to prevent goiter.)

MAKE SMART SHOPPING SECOND NATURE

I know this is going to sound counterintuitive as I'm ramping you up to get started, but I don't want you to throw away all the food in your house and start over. Eat what you have so you don't waste food. Or, if you can afford it, donate your unopened food to a local food bank so your old pantry doesn't go to waste. When your old stuff is gone, replenish with whole healthy foods and start anew.

When you shop in the grocery store, get in the habit of picking up these six things: sacks of whole-grain rice, a couple of fresh or frozen green vegetables like broccoli, kale, or spinach (and an onion, though not green, is versatile), a sweet potato or yam, some low-sodium or no-salt-added chicken or vegetable broth, your favorite protein (lean meat, fish, or tofu), and iodized salt. Then splurge on a simple sauce that is not too heavy on sugar or corn syrup, like a salsa or a coconut curry. Ideally, find sauces with no sugars—that's hard to do. Or make your own sauce if you have time. With this shopping list complete, you have all you need for a high-fiber, complex-carbohydrate dish that will provide several lunches and dinners and cost less than a few bucks a meal. Once you get this stable of go-tos down, expand your repertoire and throw in cauliflower, chard, broccoli rabe, bok choy, or whatever looks interesting. Go shopping today!

- Start in produce: sweet potatoes, pre-washed kale or spinach, sweet and red onion, fresh lime, bananas, and whatever else looks tasty
- Head to dry goods: pack of whole-wheat/whole-grain noodles, loaf of whole-wheat bread, jar of nut butter—peanut, almond, whatever looks good to you—and low-sugar jars of salsa or sauces

- Followed by the frozen section: an assortment of vegetables and fruits (if you're going to make smoothies)
- Next, the meat counter: fresh ground turkey or chicken, or whatever kind of fish or shrimp appeals to you
- Lastly, the dairy aisle: nonfat, high-protein yogurt or kefir, nonfat cow's milk, or any nut-based or oat milk

Here are some quick steps to making a balanced bowl.

1. Pour 1 cup broth and 1 cup rice into a pressure cooker, seal the device, and push the Start button.

2. While your rice is cooking, chop some vegetables, throw them into a skillet, add a protein of your choice, and sauté together with your sauce.

3. Once the rice and the veggie mixture are finished, toss them together in a bowl and enjoy. (That 1 cup rice should yield two servings.)

REPLACE CHEAT DAYS WITH REWARD DAYS

I'm not a fan of what many call the cheat day. Studies suggest it takes up to three months to effect healthier habits, whether eating better or exercising more. If you're going to make this healthy lifestyle change—if this is your time to totally upgrade the way you live—stick to a hard-core program for three months. Don't cheat, don't lie to yourself, don't sneak stuff. Own your destiny for three months, then see how you feel at the end. You will be so proud of yourself and so happy with how great you feel and how good you look, you won't want a cheat day. Then, when you consume a cheeseburger, fries, and a frothy pint again, they likely won't taste good. Or you'll take a few bites and say *Meh*.

Reward days, on the other hand, are more positive. What most men find is that the deeper they get into a healthy, low-calorie, whole-food diet, the less they want to cheat; if they avoid an unhealthy item for a few months, the craving goes away. And if they do indulge, they won't feel that great because their bodies will have become so tuned to small, energy- and nutrient-dense meals that pizza and a few beers won't sit well. That said, yes, you can still indulge in your favorite foods from time to time, and it may even provide a psychological boost. Just develop some better habits first. Need motivation? Simply ask yourself: *How do I want to live? How do I want to look? How do I want to feel?*

TIMING IS EVERYTHING

The most common meal-timing mistake I see men make is eating too late. Late meals or snacks don't leave enough time to burn those calories. They disrupt your sleep. And they likely increase your chance of acid reflux: when you lie down, food and booze can creep back up, along with acid from your stomach, and burn a hole in your throat. It doesn't happen overnight, but over years it can certainly turn into a problem. Reflux can cause pain, chronic cough, sleep problems—and sometimes cancer. Aim to stop eating within two hours of your bedtime; if you must have food in the evening, eat light and healthfully. A great light meal choice is whole-grain toast with a smear of nut butter. This gives you a little fat, a little protein, and some fiber-rich carbohydrate to sustain you until morning.

Breakfast: Less Important Than You Thought

The myth about breakfast being the most important meal of the day has persisted for decades. This idea originated as a marketing strategy by breakfast food companies in the early 1900s, and even today no good scientific studies support the breakfast myth. The reality is that no meal is more important than another; there is nothing metabolically special

Experiment with Fasting

Some pretty compelling studies say intermittent fasting is healthy, perhaps increasing longevity (or maybe it seems that way since time passes so slowly when you're hungry!). The concept of intermittent fasting goes back about 60 years in the nutrition literature. The idea, and there are many variations, is to eat zero calories for 16 hours of the day; you just drink water, coffee, or tea with no additives. Then you consume your day's calories in the 8-hour window when you break your fast. Eventually, your stomach shrinks, your entire dietary hormone profile changes, and you get used to eating in a limited time frame each day. But proceed with caution if you do heavy exercise. If you're up early and try to exercise rigorously on an empty stomach, you won't get in as good a workout. A light workout on an empty stomach followed by breakfast will give you just the right amount of energy without packing in too many calories.

Fasting is the perfect example of how to individualize your nutrition plans. If you are trying to lose weight rapidly and still eat a balanced diet of proteins, vegetables, and whole grains, intermittent fasting may be a great choice. If you are training for a marathon, body-building competition, or other athletically demanding endeavor, this is likely not the diet for you.

about breakfast. Whether you skip it or eat it should depend solely on your lifestyle. If you get up early and work out, then you should eat breakfast; otherwise your workout will suck and you'll feel miserable. If, however, you get up and head straight to work, it's okay to skip the morning meal. Instead, eat when you feel hungry. It is that simple. In fact, if you eat dinner late—say nine o'clock or later—and you get up at six, you probably *should* skip breakfast because you're likely still digesting your evening meal.

BEWARE: BREAD, YOGURT, SMOOTHIES

There's nothing more demoralizing than trying to lose weight and failing. Often, it's because you're hanging out with false friends, like bread, yogurt, and smoothies.

Bread We all know by now that white bread is out: consuming white bread is like eating sugar. But it may be time to rethink multigrain. Go to your local natural foods store and check out the labels of a half-dozen multigrain breads. Now count how many of those have *whole-wheat flour* listed as the first ingredient. It won't be many. Most multigrain breads use enriched wheat flour, which is the same as white bread. Baking birdseed into your bread and calling it multigrain doesn't make it healthy. Sure, the birdseed has some fiber, and the resulting loaf is a little better than white bread, but without the whole wheat you're not getting the fiber or metabolic benefit of real whole-grain bread. The only bread you should eat is made with 100 percent whole-grain flour.

Yogurt Yogurt has become one of the most difficult foods to decipher. In its purest form, it is an incredibly important food, packed with protein and probiotics. I *love* yogurt—I eat nonfat, no-sugar-added Icelandic or Bulgarian yogurt every day in my smoothie or with fresh blueberries. But to mask the sour taste, many "healthy" yogurts contain more sugar than a candy bar. Guys, yogurt is *supposed* to be sour, and you should either embrace its natural flavor or avoid it altogether.

Smoothies Smoothies are not created equal. Most smoothies are dietary Trojan horses, full of sugar and fat hidden behind a healthy facade. A yogurt drink from Jamba Juice actually has more calories than a stick of butter (840 versus 810). While very few men can eat a stick of butter at one sitting, just about anyone, including a child, can down a sweet, creamy fruit drink.

Made right, however—which usually means made at home—smoothies are a great way to get lots of fiber, green vegetables, healthy protein, calcium, and just enough calories to keep you going for the day. A good smoothie should have no fruit juice—I repeat, *no fruit juice*! A good smoothie *should* contain whole fruits (fresh or frozen), protein (like no-sugar-added peanut butter, other nut butters, powdered protein, or high-protein nonfat yogurt), a fiber with healthy fats (like chia seed or flaxseed), and any nonfat non-sweetened milk (cow, nut, soy, or oat—doesn't matter). That is it. *No* immunity boosts or serenity boosts or energy boosts, or whatever other mythical concoctions.

Here's my go-to smoothie most mornings:

1 cup (235 ml) milk

2 tablespoons sugar-free, fat-free high-protein
   yogurt (Greek, Icelandic, or Bulgarian)

1 banana

1½ tablespoons peanut butter powder

1½ tablespoons flaxseed

Handful fresh spinach or kale

1 cup (135 g) fruit, like strawberries or blueberries

Place all ingredients in a blender with about 5 ice cubes. Blend it to your desired consistency and go.

"GOOD" FATS VERSUS "BAD" FATS

Let me tell you, I could explain the differences between good and bad fats, but the nutritional science is conflicting on this topic, and there are entrenched camps proclaiming how important a type of fat consumption is. What everyone agrees on is that our bodies—and especially the brain—need some fat for normal function. Calorically, however, fat is superdense, so eating more fat than you need will cause you to take in too many calories, and you'll store those extra calories as body fat. Personally, I don't think the *kind* of fat you eat is as important as the *amount* of fat you consume (unless you have severe coronary disease, in which case you need to follow a strict prescription diet your nutritionist or cardiologist designs for you). For most guys, I recommend you simply know the difference between unsaturated (the "good" fats), saturated, and trans fats:

Unsaturated Fats

- Found in plants and nuts
- Are liquid at room temperature, most commonly sold as vegetable oils

- Come in two forms, monounsaturated and polyunsaturated. (Some studies show that polyunsaturated fats may be a bit better for your heart, but you'd have to make fat consumption part of an overall healthy, reduced-calorie lifestyle to see the benefits. In other words, if you ate a quart of olive oil a day because it's a healthy fat, you're eating too much of a good thing.) Tree nuts are great sources of polyunsaturated fats—walnuts, almonds, Brazil nuts.

Saturated Fats

- Found in animal products, including butter, and some plants, like palm and coconut
- Are solid at room temperature, like coconut oil
- Saturated fats have been vilified by many nutritionists and scientists as potentially increasing the risk of cholesterol plaque formation and worsening risk for heart attack. Saturated fats have just as many calories as unsaturated fats, and foods rich in saturated fat, like hamburgers, are easier to eat in large portions versus foods rich in unsaturated fats, like nuts. You would have to eat more than a cup of almonds to approach the same number of fat calories found in a third-pound 85 percent lean hamburger. The science of whether it's actually the saturated fat that is intrinsically more harmful than unsaturated fat is pretty flimsy. Moderation is key.

Trans Fats

- Not found in nature
- Are called trans fats because chemists figured out how to turn an unsaturated fat into a saturated fat. Best example: margarine. Why mess with nature like this? Because of bad science. Years ago, studies came out showing that dietary saturated fats caused more coronary plaque buildup than unsaturated fats. Coronary plaque buildup leads to heart disease. So some clever chemists figured if they could add hydrogen molecules to vegetable oil, people could put "healthy butter" on their toast. Wrong. Turns out the body can't recognize trans fats and thus treats them like saturated fats, and you still get coronary plaque buildup. Trans fats may be even worse than saturated fats. Whoops.

EATING BY THE DECADES

As you get older, the rules change. If you're 40 and still eating like you're 20, you're in for a rude awakening.

Teens

You're still growing and can pretty much eat whatever you want without too many consequences. Sure, adolescent obesity is on the rise and boys can override their caloric growth demands, but, for the most part, you can get away with a lot of ice cream as a teenager—especially as an active teenager.

20s

Things are starting to get real here. If you left home to go to college, you have open access to food, sometimes banquet, trough-style dorm buffets. Your parents aren't making food decisions for you anymore, and you may be under a lot of academic stress. But this is your decade to set yourself up for a lifetime of good habits. Practice calorie restriction; don't go back for seconds at the dorm trough.

30s

For many men, this is a tough decade. Your career is taking off, you may have a partner and a mortgage and possibly even children. All of these take time, and you may neglect your nutrition. If you're a dad, don't finish your kid's mac and cheese. Commit to setting an example for yourself and your family by following a healthy, whole-food eating plan.

40s

Now your metabolism is starting to slow down as part of the aging process. This is the decade to reduce your caloric consumption or the weight *will* creep up on you. Even if you remain active, you *still* will likely want to cut back. Remember that your testosterone levels may start dropping, too, which can slow your metabolism—so get a testosterone blood test if you are packing on weight and don't think your diet has changed.

50s

This decade will be a continuation of your 40s—keep eating less, exercising more. As you age, the intensity of your workouts likely goes down, so eat smarter and less to accommodate this change.

60s

As men age, bone density declines due to less activity and lower testosterone levels. Make sure you're supplementing your vitamin D and calcium levels either by taking supplements or by upping dietary calcium to 500 milligrams a day of calcium citrate. Boost your vitamin D naturally by getting 10 to 15 minutes of sun exposure with 30 SPF sunscreen.

70s

Later in life, it's harder to keep on muscle mass. Now, more than ever, good protein is important. You may consider adding a protein shake with 30 to 60 grams of protein to your diet. Any protein source is fine: whey, pea, soy (I don't get fussed about men taking in a little soy protein—too much soy may lead to lower testosterone levels, but not at these doses).

80s and beyond

If you are still healthy at 80, congratulations! Your good genes and healthy lifestyle have let you live this long. Keeping your lean protein up for good muscle mass and eating lots of green leafy veggies and whole grains will keep your digestive health optimal. But if you want a little cake and ice cream, go for it! You won the game.

SMART SNACKING

Despite what we're told, snacking is not a bad thing if you're snacking with healthy purpose. In fact, snacking can be the key to healthy eating. Eating multiple small meals throughout the day is a good, disciplined way to not feel hungry and get great nutrition. But small meals should be protein-dense, like a handful of nuts, or fiber-dense, like a whole-grain cracker with nut butter. That said, snacking can take you down a dark road if you're doing it to relieve stress. Stress depletes your reward hormone, dopamine. Food quickly raises dopamine levels. When dopamine levels are low, you feel tired, even depressed and not motivated. Your body craves a dopamine rush. If you're trying to lose weight, you have to resist the urge to snack on sugary, salty foods. Take three deep breaths in through the nose and exhale through your mouth *before* you grab that chocolate bar. Here are two other tools for smarter snacking:

Mind over Cracker

The next time you feel that familiar anxious pit in your stomach, acknowledge it. Feel it for what it is— stress, not hunger—and take a few deep breaths. Awareness will help you power through. Perhaps drink a glass of water or a cup of black coffee or tea. The act of drinking alone can distract you from wanting to eat long enough to get your dopamine from another source, like a quick walk or workout. Or send a text to your partner, maybe something sexy to get your mind out of the kitchen and into the bedroom.

Keep Nuts Nearby

First of all, let's get one thing clear: a peanut is not a nut. It's a bean, or a legume, and its nutritional properties are closer to beans than tree nuts. While peanuts have good protein levels and a decent vitamin profile, they also have quite a few carbohydrates. Real nuts, however, are perhaps the greatest snack on the planet. Among the most powerful and nutrient-packed varieties are Brazil nuts, almonds, walnuts, pecans, and macadamia nuts—they are full of healthy polyunsaturated fats, which are heart healthy *and* sperm healthy. These nuts also contain a lot of calories, so if you're trying to lose weight, keep your nuts to a handful a day (yeah, I know how that sounds) until you've lost the weight and are eating better in general. Cashews, pistachios, and hazelnuts are great, too, but they have even *more* carbohydrates, so weight watchers beware.

MULTIVITAMINS ARE NO BETTER THAN A GOOD MEAL

A multivitamin will not harm you. But if you eat whole foods with lots of fruits and vegetables in all colors of the rainbow—such as leafy greens, orange carrots, red beets, purple grapes—you'll get all the vitamins you need. If you do splurge, a once-a-day men's vitamin is plenty.

Hydration Education

Believe it or not, there's a good chance you're overhydrated. You probably never expected a doctor to tell you to drink less water—a urologist, no less, who regularly treats kidney stones (a common problem with chronically dehydrated people). But most people who mind their health by taking advice from magazines, fitness blogs, or Instagram influencers get the message that they don't drink enough water. Many so-called health experts suggest you drink way more water than you need. Look no further than the soft drink industry to find the source of this bad advice. Fifteen years ago, Americans dramatically cut back on soda consumption because, well, we finally realized how bad it was. But we're brand conscious and like walking around with French and Polynesian water labels. With no real data from real doctors or real science, the bottled-water industry told us we were pathologically thirsty. Yes, good hydration is a pillar of good health; it promotes kidney health, aids in weight loss, optimizes exercise, and does all kinds of other wonderful things. But optimal hydration is different for everyone, and many men simply drink too much water. Overhydration can cause low sodium levels, frequent urination (duh), and even seizures and death if you really overdo it.

DRINK WHEN YOU ARE THIRSTY—IT'S THAT SIMPLE

Your water needs depend on how active you are and how much fat versus lean weight you carry. So you're not going to get a recommendation from me on how many ounces a day you should drink. I have no idea how much I drink. I work out a lot, sweat a lot, and drink a lot of water; that's about as scientific as I get. Trust your body on this one. When you're thirsty, drink.

I see a lot of men in my clinic who ignore their thirst. Men who fight Los Angeles traffic every day don't want to get caught on the 405 Freeway with a full bladder. Busy guys who run from meeting to meeting may not carry water with them and thus wait to drink until they get home at night. **How do you know how much water to drink? Simple: drink when you're thirsty, and never ignore thirst.** Our bodies are so in tune to water balance—we have many biochemical and hormonal mechanisms in the brain and the kidneys to regulate water intake; thirst dictates our water needs. If you exercise a lot or live in the desert, you'll get thirsty more often, and you should drink more water. Another surefire way to make sure you're drinking enough water is to look at your pee. If it's dark yellow or orange, you need to drink more H_2O (a lot more). If your urine is yellow to pale yellow, you're just right. If it's clear, you may be overhydrated (don't worry, your body can usually sense when it's overhydrated, and you'll just pee more). You definitely do not need to drink bottled water—invest in a filter and a reusable water bottle. Plus, it's pretty much socially unacceptable these days to have a plastic water bottle. All the cool kids are drinking out of a glass or recycled aluminum canister.

SAY GOODBYE TO SODA (IF YOU CAN)

Or, pop, for you Midwesterners. The easy answer to a man's soda dilemma—to drink or not to drink—is *not* to drink. I know, I have a soft spot for the stuff, too. But there is no health reason to drink soda. I'm sure you already knew that, but if you needed a doctor to tell you, I'm telling you now. I will say this, though: artificial sweeteners have been around for decades, and not one death has been attributed to them. I also don't buy the notion that they trick your body and make you fatter—there is no data for that. But just like with alcohol or any other vice, moderation is key. I admit that I drink a diet cola now and again. My kids give me grief, as they don't drink the stuff, but I do like the fizz and taste. Sparkling waters are almost as good, and those are definitely my first go-tos.

CAFFEINE CAN BE GOOD FOR YOU

Caffeine is a chemical in the class of methylxanthines, a stimulant that increases release of ATP (adenosine triphosphate) from the cell membrane. ATP accelerates heart rate, increases neurotransmitter release to increase alertness. It's addictive. And your body builds a tolerance—the more you consume, the more you crave. It's found naturally in tea, coffee, chocolate, and kola berry and is water soluble. Translating that science into clear language—caffeine makes a super energy drink, and a multi-billion-dollar legal market.

Coffee

I love my espresso and drink about four cups a day—two in the morning and one or two around three p.m. Many nutritional experts will say that's terrible, but it works for me and my lifestyle. And it turns out there is strong science outlining real benefits of coffee beans aside from that inimitable caffeine boost we crave. For one, coffee is packed with antioxidants, which fight inflammation (other foods, of course, provide antioxidants, like leafy green vegetables, dark berries, and grapes). Second, pretty good studies show that two to four cups of coffee a day reduces the risk of dementia, diabetes, and depression (three Ds you don't want). Moderate coffee intake—that is, fewer than four cups a day—also may improve sperm function for all the aspiring dads in the audience.

That said, coffee curbs appetite, which could help you lose weight *or* throw off a balanced diet, depending on who you are. And if you have heart arrhythmias, coffee can definitely make those rhythm problems worse (check with your doctor). Moderation is key. Eight cups of coffee a day is probably an indication you're burning it too hard. Bottom line, if you don't like the taste of coffee, and never developed the habit, don't force yourself to drink it. If you do drink it, don't drink too much.

Tea

Tea contains caffeine, too. Not as much per glass or cup as coffee, but caffeine is caffeine. Apply the same rule of consuming fewer than four cups a day. Tea drinking, of course, is significant as a social time in many cultures. I'm all in favor of taking a break for any reason (other than a smoke break) during a busy day.

Energy Drinks

These should be a last resort because most of them are packed with sugar and supplements you don't need. Instead, down a cup of black coffee. You'll get the same energy boost without pumping yourself full of additional vitamins, sugars, colorings, and other unpronounceable additives. If you need the kick and can't tolerate coffee or tea, fine, have an energy drink. But please, make it a sugar-free one.

PROCEED WITH CAUTION

Sports Drinks

If you're looking to replenish essential nutrients you may have lost during a workout, sports drinks are the *last* thing you should drink. There's *a lot* of crap in them: sugar, fake sugar, a ton of vitamins and minerals you *don't* need, and more sugar (oh, and there's the plastic). Unless you're sweating hard for 30-plus minutes during a workout, you do not need electrolytes. If, on the other hand, you do sweat a great deal when you exercise, by all means, add a little sugar-free electrolyte solution to your water.

There are some good electrolyte solutions that have no sugar or artificial sweeteners. I'm always going to tell you to keep it simple, to avoid any additives you can, but synthetic sweeteners, in moderation, won't kill you. Medical science has over 50 years of pretty good data that you'd have to drink gallons of fake sugar drinks a day to potentially harm yourself. But again, you can avoid fake sugar altogether and still get a good electrolyte solution. Nuun tablets are a favorite of mine—no sugar, and a bit bitter, but they do add some natural flavors to offset.

ENJOY ALCOHOL, BUT UNDERSTAND IT

I get asked all the time whether one or two glasses of wine or beer a day is okay. Alcohol is celebratory; it's fun, relaxing, and social and has been part of human society for thousands of years, so I get the cultural significance and would not want to interfere with a good party—parties relieve stress and stress is bad. But let's be clear: alcohol is poison, plain and simple. Thankfully, it is a poison your body can break down easily, so long as it is consumed in small quantities. Alcohol quickly becomes harmful if you drink too much. If you are able to limit your alcohol intake to, say, one or max two drinks at a sitting, you'll be fine.

But here are other ways alcohol can be harmful. Alcohol is loaded with calories—wasted calories that are worse than sugar (alcohol is almost twice as calorically dense as sugar). For anyone who needs to lose weight, there is no place for alcohol in the diet. None. If you're trying to make a baby, any more than one or two drinks per day kills sperm. If you and your partner have been trying to conceive for over six months and not succeeding, stop drinking altogether and see a fertility specialist.

Chapter Cheat Sheet

☐ Weight loss can be easy; don't eat so much.

☐ Diets don't work—changing your relationship with food does.

☐ Keep your shopping simple: whole grains, green vegetables, fruit, lean meats, and nonfat dairy are key.

☐ A few kitchen essentials, such as a good blender and a pressure cooker, are all you need to cook great meals at home.

☐ Drink when you're thirsty.

☐ Eat the rainbow of veggies and fruits to get your vitamins and micronutrients.

☐ Drink caffeine in moderation.

☐ Easy on the booze.

04

MOVE

A Man's Guide to Strength and Fitness

Exercise shouldn't be complicated. Given my thoughts on diets (see page 80), it's probably no surprise that I'm not a big fan of elaborate exercise plans either. **If you decide to move more today than you did yesterday, that's an exercise plan.** If you decide to walk, you have a plan (or if you can't walk, a physical therapy program is a plan). What I want to see from you is a minor initial change in your exercise habits. When you have an extra 30 minutes, don't write it off as too little time to walk, go to the gym, or hop in the pool. If you can do 10 pushups today, try 11 tomorrow, 12 the next day, maybe a hundred on day 50, then just keep going. If you can walk up two flights of stairs today, walk up three tomorrow, and four the next day. If you live or work in a 20-story building, you have a free gym, step by step.

Sorry, there are no shortcuts to living a healthier life. If you want to look and feel amazing, you're going to have to dedicate part of each day to exercise. But be realistic—and go easy on yourself. Sure, we can all strive for a perfect Hollywood body and feel great if we achieve that goal. But we should also know how hard that is to do. It requires a lot of sacrifice, and it's difficult to maintain while still finding time for the joy in life we get from sharing meals with friends and not spending our entire lives in the gym. The truth about those Hollywood bodies is that, with few exceptions, they don't stay Hollywood bodies when filming ends. What you see on camera is *not* how that guy looks all year long. More important, there's no science that says washboard abs help you live longer or make you happier. Lots of science, however, says that simply working out four or five times a week will improve longevity, make your heart healthier, reduce your risk of cancer, and, you bet, boost your sex life. You'll feel better, and you will live longer.

Overcoming Mental Hurdles

Check the ego, be vulnerable, and prepare to fail. Your journey to becoming a healthy man will require help at first. You're not going to hear me say "You got this" because, right now, you probably don't. But you *will* get this, for sure. You just have to stop fronting and start realizing it's hard to make change and be healthy and better. Never forget: all it takes is *a little more than the day before*.

SET REALISTIC EXPECTATIONS

Imagine it's December 31 and you're planning to start your exercise program January 1. You set your alarm for five a.m.—you normally get up at seven—and hit the gym for an hour. If you can keep up this regimen for the next few months, that's amazing. I love hearing about people who transform their lives by *radically* changing their lifestyle. But it's not realistic for most of us. For most of us, the wheels come off after a couple of weeks of pre-dawn gym workouts. All it takes is one night where you stayed up a bit late and couldn't get out of bed the next day—you skip the gym one day, then it's easier to skip the next and the next, and before long the wheels are off and you're not exercising at all. Why do that to yourself? You've added guilt and stress to what was supposed to be a life-changing, uplifting experience. This isn't meant to be bummer material. I want you to be realistic with yourself. If you start off racing out of the gate, you lose steam. You can still live well and feel great by exercising as little as 30 minutes a day, five days a week. But it has to be high-quality, high-heart-rate activity. Walking, gardening, or doing housework is better than nothing, but you should be breathless while you're exercising. The more calories you burn, the more often your body goes into fat deficit. I want you to make gradual changes—a little every day to reset yourself.

COACH MACK, 48

One Small Step for a Man . . .

When I was in high school, Coach Mack managed my baseball team. After summer break one year, Coach Mack swaggered back on campus about 50 pounds lighter than when our season ended in spring. All the players were shocked at how great Big Mack looked. When asked what he did, he said it was simple: when school ended, he hit rock bottom with how he looked and felt. He was embarrassed that he was an athletic coach and was so heavy. He waited for summer so no one would see him and went to the school track every day. The first day, he couldn't make a quarter-mile lap without stopping and gasping for air. By the end of the first week, he easily had a quarter mile, and every day after that, he went a little farther than the day before. By end of summer, he was walking and jogging three miles, and it got easier every day—a little more than the day before.

ENOUGH WITH THE EXCUSES

When I see a man in my clinic whom I haven't seen for a while, and I notice he's put on weight, I always ask him, "What's going on? What happened?" Far too often the excuses are worryingly hollow. Him: "Well, I hurt my knee, so I couldn't exercise anymore." Me: "You still have two arms and one good leg. Get in the pool, get on a rower, get into physical therapy to build up that knee." *I hurt my knee?* Try losing a leg or two and still be a competitive athlete like some of our Paralympians. If this kind of excuse sounds familiar, face it: you don't have the mindset yet to overcome minor adversity to live a more active lifestyle. But you will. That's why you're here. You want to get it; you want to change (or at least the person who gave you this book wants you to change). If you have an injury, you have to adapt. A shoulder injury may mean no tennis for a while, but you can still jog, walk fast, maybe bike. A knee or hip injury may mean more upper-body-heavy workouts or, if you have access to a pool, swim. **There's always something you can do.**

FITTING IT ALL IN

Most of us work an eight-hour day, five days a week (or more). Do not ignore healthy habits during this time. If you have an hour lunch, get at least a little fitness in: walk, do stairs in your building, anything. No need to buy an expensive standing desk—they don't make much of a difference and probably aren't good for your posture. Instead, make sure you're simply getting up and moving around for at least five minutes every hour.

Whatever fitness approach you take, stay hydrated, especially if you plan to work out in the evening, by sipping water every hour after lunch to preload for an evening run or fitness class (but don't overhydrate; see page 112). I work out at about six o'clock most nights, so I make sure to eat a snack and drink a cup of coffee around 3:30. This routine gives me great energy levels to get a fantastic workout in. I get home around eight and have a light supper.

> **A CALL TO ACTION** If you cannot do ten push-ups or walk up two flights of stairs without stopping and gasping for air, you need a change. You should also see a physician to check your heart function before beginning any serious exercise. My primary goal for men is to help them make sure they never get to a place in which they can't possibly imagine getting back into shape. The worst deal with falling apart is having to put yourself back together. The muscle fatigue, tiredness, and soreness that strike during that first week of workouts are motivation enough for me never to stray too far from my ideal fitness level.

A READY-MADE ROUTINE

Many psychology and human behavioral studies suggest it takes three months of dedicated effort to engrain a new behavior as a habit. The following simple one-week routine, no gym or equipment needed, that includes cardio and strength training, can be repeated for the entire first three months of your journey to becoming a healthier man. Your body will tell you when it is ready to take on more distance, add more reps, and increase your heart rate. You should start ramping up the minute you feel up to it. Also, don't take many days off and always fall back to this baseline workout. As with any new health routine, check with your doctor to make sure you're fit for this. The good thing is, this routine is self-paced so you can advance when you're ready. Most important, mix it up and have fun.

Day 1

- Walk 7,000 to 10,000 steps—all at once if you can or break it up into 2 sessions.
- Do as many push-ups as you can, whether it's 2 or 50, then rest for 30 seconds and repeat. Do that six times.
- Do as many air squats as you can. Start in a standing position, arms at your side, feet shoulder-width apart. Swing your arms straight out as you bend your knees until your thighs are parallel to the floor, then pop back up. Wait 30 seconds, then repeat three times.

Day 2

- Walk 7,000 to 10,000 steps but *faster* than you did yesterday; maybe even jog a bit.
- If you're not too sore, repeat the push-ups and squats.
- Add front and side planks (see page 137). For the plank, hold yourself in the up position of a push-up and hold until you collapse; wait 30 seconds and go to a left-side plank, then hold it until you fail; wait 30 seconds and go to a right plank. Do six sets of planks or as many as you can before fatigue sets in.

Day 3

- Walk 10,000 steps.
- Add 20 minutes of intense cardio activity (anything to get your heart rate up to 80 percent of max for the entire 20 minutes; see page 130).

Day 4

- Walk 5,000 to 10,000 steps (no extra cardio or resistance today).

Day 5

- Walk 10,000 steps.
- Add 20 minutes of intense cardio.
- Complete the entire push-up and air squat resistance program from day 1.

Day 6

- Walk 10,000 steps.
- Repeat the resistance program from day 2.

Day 7

- Walk 10,000 or more steps, then rest.

HIRE A PRO

If you want to get strong but don't have much weight-lifting experience, hire a trainer to walk you through the basic moves and form. I've been lifting since I was 11 and borrowed my older brother's weights, and I get that not everyone has the depth of experience to start a weight program without oversight. I see too many guys repping out with *horrible* form and wasting their time and risking injury. If you're superserious about making gains, staying injury-free, and even getting a little extra nutrition advice, trainers can help you there, too. All you probably need are a few sessions to learn some fundamentals and check in with your trainer periodically as you make additional gains. These people are pros who can accelerate the fitness process and keep you superfocused.

FITNESS BY THE DECADES

Will the workout you do in your 20s still work in your 50s? While the principles remain the same no matter what age you are, what I might recommend to a 20-year-old patient is certainly different from what I recommend to an 80-year-old. It can be empowering to understand how age may influence your exercise routine. No matter how many years you have under your belt, your best strategy is to always fall back to the basics: eat less than you did yesterday, move more than you did yesterday, and sleep better than you did yesterday.

20s

This is the decade to pack on muscle and prime your heart. Heart cholesterol plaques start forming in adolescence, which lead to heart disease later in life. If you get your heart rate up to 80 percent of your target max—for a 20-year-old, that's in the 160s—for at least 30 minutes a day, you will set yourself up for a great adulthood.

Testosterone levels start declining after age 25, and vigorous exercise in your 20s will maintain your T levels as you get older. One of the first signs of molecular aging, loss of high nitric oxide levels, starts between ages 25 and 28. As poet Dylan Thomas admonished, rage against the dying of the light!

30s

Let's hope you've established a great foundation in your 20s because, most likely, you'll be professionally and personally busier in your 30s. If you don't have a great foundation, welcome! The good news is, it only takes a few months to build that new foundation of better nutrition, higher level of exercise, and better sleep habits. This will prepare you for taking on the joy and stressors of life in your 30s—you may be married, starting a family, and accelerating your career. These things are awesome, but they are demanding and stressful. You'll want to use exercise as an escape and stress reliever even as you maintain strong testosterone levels, bone density, and heart health. Couples workouts are a great way to bond with your partner—studies show that couples who exercise together are happier, more sexual, and more grounded. Working out single may open you up to meeting someone on a trail, in a gym, or pursuing like-minded fitness activities.

40s

This is where many men start to feel their age. Our joints and muscles do take longer to recover, we get stiffer, and we are more prone to injury. If you're starting an exercise program in your 40s, take it slow. Instead of exercising hard five to seven days a week, maybe start at three to five days a week and work your way up. This gives your joints a chance to catch up to your eager brain and willing muscles. Don't make excuses for your age; embrace your wisdom, and the first time you pass a younger guy on the trail, take pride.

50s

Exercise prevents cancer. If for no other reason, stay fit in this decade so you can be there for your grandkids. Listen to your body, but don't be afraid to push yourself a little past your comfort zone. A little soreness is fine, especially when you haven't put in the time recently. Keep moving and the soreness will go away. Vigorous exercise in your 50s will prevent bone and muscle loss and keep your heart healthy. Vigorous exercise for a man in his 50s should be 30 minutes a day at 80 percent of your max heart rate—somewhere in the 140s to 150s, and higher as you get in better shape. A jog or run is vigorous. Moving through a weight-lifting circuit for 30 minutes certainly counts. Any activity that makes it tough for you to carry on a conversation is vigorous.

60s

There are tons of 60-plus men running marathons, power lifting, swimming the English Channel, and climbing mountains—there's no reason that can't be you. (Unless you don't want it to be you!) Those endeavors take time and money and sacrifice, but these guys should serve as reminders that you can most likely be superactive and superfit and still retain your day job. Keep your partner's fitness up as well—it's good for relationships and good for lowering depression risk. An interesting thing happens to the heart as we age: it actually develops more blood vessels (a process known as neovascularization), which is why a guy in his 60s has a better chance of surviving a heart attack than a guy in his 40s. But please, proceed in your fitness regimen with caution—and expert advice—especially if you have a history of heart disease.

70s and Beyond

You should at least be walking daily, for as many steps as you can, and you can probably do some weightlifting as well. Resistance training late in life improves bone density, muscle mass, and mood. Men with neurological disorders like Parkinson's disease benefit a lot from weight-bearing exercise. The rule of muscle building in your 70s is light resistance: start with five- or ten-pound weights and work through simple range-of-motion exercises like arm curls, shoulder presses, and bench presses to activate skeletal muscle building. Make sure you know your testosterone levels and consider replacement therapy (see page 43) to keep your bone health strong and your sexual health optimized. Vigorous exercise in your 70s, 80s, and beyond will help maintain these things. Your definition of vigorous exercise changes as you age—a brisk walk, swimming laps in a pool, or even lifting weights works at your age.

GET A DOG

Hear me out on this one: dogs can play a huge part in our well-being (cats, too, I suppose, but try jogging on the beach with your cat). Taking care of a dog is good for your soul, good for your blood pressure, good for teaching kids, if you have them, some responsibility. Best of all, dogs *love* exercise— walking, running, you name it. It's hard not to be more active when you own a dog. My day starts at five or six a.m. with a brisk walk with my black standard poodle. He's typically a late sleeper (loves weekends) but still pops up every morning, tail wagging, and does a full-body stretch before our predawn walk. Afterward, he goes back to sleep and I go to work (not a bad life being my dog). Once I get home from work, the whole family takes him for a long walk after dinner (our last chance to hit our daily 10,000-step goal).

WHAT'S A DAD SUPPOSED TO DO TO GET IN SHAPE?

Exercise takes time. If you have a family, especially young children, you may think working out takes time away from them. It doesn't have to. When I was a young dad, I purchased a jogging stroller, strapped my toddler in, ran five miles to a playground. While we played at the playground, I rehydrated and ate a snack; 30 minutes later, I ran the five miles home. You can modify that regimen to accommodate your fitness level. When that toddler started high school and joined the football team, we both got up before five a.m., went to the gym, and worked out for an hour. I dropped him off at school and I went into the hospital. Great workout, great family time. By the time he was a sophomore, he was crushing me in everything from bench press max to squats. Despite my insanely competitive nature, nothing made me prouder. Now that his college football career is over, he still works out like crazy. I'd like to think his early fitness exposure with his dad created a lifelong habit of staying in shape.

Now that I'm 50, I'm not putting up heavy weights in the gym, but I'm still keeping in shape with my family. My younger son, now in high school, challenges me to weekly fitness competitions to see who can burn the most calories in a week. We run, lift weights, do stationary bikes and rowing machines. On days when I don't want to test my limits, he pushes me on—or shames me. Point is, unless you're training for an Ironman or marathon, you can get your kids involved and teach them the importance of regular exercise.

Set an example. Your children will look at you and up to you. If you're hitting it hard to stay in shape, so will they.

HAVE FUN WITH FITNESS TRACKERS

Fitness gadgets are everywhere, but do you need one to get fit? I don't endorse specific brands, but I do think a smart watch or a bracelet that counts your steps and tracks your heart rate is a great investment. Fitness tracking motivates and keeps you honest. A fitness tracker tells me that if I didn't burn 800 calories over my resting calorie consumption, I have to step it up before I go to bed (the dog gets an extra walk, or I have to squeeze in a workout). Obsessive? Maybe. But I think it can be fun to hold yourself accountable. The only wearable that is all but essential is a simple heart rate monitor (either chest straps or bracelets; both are accurate). I also like step counters. You can get an all-in-one watch that tracks both steps and heart rate. You never truly know how hard you're working or whether you're making progress unless you have some metrics. Fitness trackers are also a great way for you to look back and see how far you've come. If you couldn't do 5,000 steps at the beginning of the month and you're striding out 10,000 by the end, rock on, brother.

PUBLIC GYMS VERSUS HOME GYMS

Gyms are fantastic places to exercise, be social, and learn new moves by watching fitness buffs grind out their workouts. For me, the gym is a mental boost, and I treat it as a reward for a full day treating patients. It's dedicated time where I try to keep phone calls as close to zero as a busy doctor can. Ear buds go in, Metallica gets cranked, and I zone out. But I get it: joining a gym is a luxury. For those who can't afford it—or want to spend their money elsewhere—thank goodness for the internet. There is so much high-quality fitness content out there these days, for both advice and routines. If you're on a tight budget, you don't need to join a gym to get into fantastic shape. Gyms can also be dirty places. Given the heightened awareness of infectious diseases since the COVID-19 pandemic, we have to make decisions about how much we want to expose ourselves. If you go to the gym, make sure you keep your distance from others and wipe down equipment before and after usage. My guess is wearing face masks in public will be with us on and off, depending on infection risk at the time. Therefore, mask up when appropriate.

If you have the space and the money to create a home gym, I say go for it. I am a huge fan of interactive fitness like Peloton and Hydrow with their curated instructor-led courses in stationary cycling and rowing. The power of having a fitness instructor streaming into your home is a marvel of technology. But these are expensive pieces of equipment with a monthly subscription fee, so I get that these luxuries are not in everyone's budget. If you can commit to the cost, go for it. While you're at it, get some dumbbells and a flat weight bench. There are all-in-one kettlebell and dumbbell sets that save space. They feature two kettlebells or two dumbbells that go up to around 40 pounds each, and you click how much weight you lift. You can click all the weight and lift the entire thing, or you can click fractions, so you lift only 20 pounds or 10 pounds at a time. These sets are pricey, but with them you don't need an entire wall rack of weights to get a solid workout at home.

The Moves

Many fitness experts, and the fitness industry as a whole, confuse the general public and make exercise seem complicated. It doesn't have to be. Here I will define and break down cardio versus resistance training. While you can't really separate the two, you can emphasize one over the other, depending on whether you're trying to lose weight or put on muscle. It's going to be simple—you won't need a gym or fancy equipment to get started and maintain a healthy exercise program.

STRENGTH AND CARDIO ARE *NOT* MUTUALLY EXCLUSIVE

Cardio workouts are those that get your heart rate up to rapid beating. (Ideally, at 80 percent of your maximum heart rate for at least 20 minutes, which will shred fat and improve your health and heart function; calculating precise max heart rate is a specific process explained on page 130.) Strength training is essentially resistance work, in which you're flexing your muscles in hopes of building bigger muscles (weightlifting being the classic example). Anytime you are using your body to perform work on a mass—whether it's with a dumbbell, kettlebell, or your own body, as with a push-up—you are doing strength training. What about yard work? Sure, raking leaves and pushing a lawnmower are good. This sounds crazy (and my wife thinks I'm crazy), but when I vacuum, I lift the canister with one hand and push the wand with the other. That's a half hour of pushing and curls, and the house looks great as well!

The new research in physiology doesn't dichotomize strength versus cardio. Hybrid workouts that mix weightlifting with cardio and boot camp–style classes are all the rage for a reason. They work. Any program that combines a session of weightlifting followed by a burst of intense cardio is a hybrid workout. For example, if you run a half mile or mile, then lift heavy weights right after while your heart rate is still high from the run, you're in a hybrid workout. Classes like CrossFit, Orangetheory Fitness, and F45 Training are great examples of hybrid workout plans.

But you do not need a class to mix it up. Traditionally, we think of things like stair walking, swimming, or running as cardio. If you're the guy at the gym who reps 12 on the bench then sits and takes selfies after your pump, you're probably working pure strength. But if you lift weights fast enough, you're also doing cardio. You can burn calories and lose fat when you do strength training. That said, it is pretty hard to drop a lot of weight because your muscles will simply fatigue before your heart rate maximizes.

If you aim to lose fat weight and put on muscle, you'll probably have to do more traditional aerobic cardio workouts like running, swimming, or cycling to maintain 80 percent of your heart rate for at least 20 minutes.

SMART WORKOUTS ARE BETTER THAN LONG WORKOUTS

If time is an issue, one really effective short workout is a high-intensity interval training (HIIT) session. These can get you into great shape in 20 minutes a day. The idea is to boost your heart rate intensely high for short bursts, with short rests in between. The higher you get your heart rate, the more calories you burn. You tend to burn fat even after your workout is finished as your heart will still be beating fast long after you walk out the gym door. A variation of HIIT is Tabata, created by Izumi Tabata, a Japanese physiologist. Tabata is a two-to-one ratio of intense activity followed by short rest: for example, 20 seconds of intensity followed by 10 seconds of rest, repeated for a total of 4 minutes. Then you take a 1- to 2-minute rest and start over. Most people can do only one or two rounds of Tabata before they're wrecked (in a good way).

There are apps you can buy that will give you effective HIIT and Tabata workouts. A classic Tabata cycle is 20 seconds of push-ups, 10 seconds of rest; 20 seconds of plank exercises, 10 seconds of rest; 20 seconds of lunges or squats, 10 seconds of rest; and 20 seconds of crunches with 10 seconds of rest. Then repeat. That gets you a crazy 4-minute cycle. You can throw in jumping jacks, burpees, whatever callisthenic you remember from gym class. I love doing Tabata workouts when I travel because I don't need a gym, and I'm usually tired and don't want to leave the hotel. But after just 8 minutes, I've done a good workout.

Classic Tabata Exercises

For a high-intensity workout, do a series of
exercises for 20 seconds each with a 10-second rest
in between. Rest for 1 to 2 minutes and repeat.

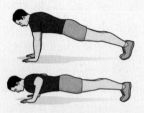

Push-Ups
As many as you can for 20
seconds, rest 10 seconds

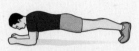

Planks
Hold for as long as you
can, rest 10 seconds

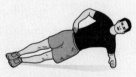

Side Planks
Hold for as long as you can,
rest 10 seconds (switch sides
on next round)

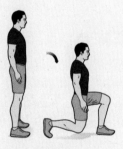

Lunges
As many as you can for
20 seconds, rest 10 seconds

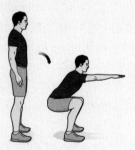

Air Squats
As many as you can for
20 seconds, rest 1 to 2 minutes
before starting over

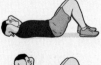
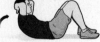

Crunches
As many as you can for
20 seconds, rest 10 seconds

TREADMILLS VERSUS TRAIL RUNS

For many men, exercising in nature connects them to some primordial flow; they need that expanse, that open space that a mountain hike or open-sea kayaking gives them. There's plenty of science to back the benefits—getting outside, breathing fresh air, and changing scenery is top-shelf medicine. But nature terrifies some guys—they don't know how to hike, what to pack, what shoes to wear, or how to follow a trail. If you're that guy, don't stress it. Stick to the treadmill and eucalyptus-infused towels. It's all good: just move.

AN ODE TO WALKING

I talk about walking your dog, getting in 10,000 or more steps, but I'd like to take a moment to single out and honor the walk. Walking is low impact but does have fitness health benefits—it's good for maintaining bone health, and body movement is excellent for gut movement and GI health. Walks aren't dramatic. You don't get your heart rate up high. But they are amazing for our souls. Walking intentionally slows the pace of a busy day. When I'm at work, running between the operating room and the office, I walk at an Olympic pace, but when I get home for the night, I walk at a leisurely pace and it feels so good. Walking is in our DNA. Even if you're wheelchair dependent for mobility, getting outside and moving is top-notch therapy. If you have a partner or partners for your walk, it's a great time to talk. If you're walking solo, it's a great time to think.

Maintenance

So you started! That's great. Maybe you've noticed some pounds coming off, maybe you're more motivated to ratchet up your fitness. I'm all for it! That's the point of starting somewhere and getting to where you are now. Now it's time to consider how you keep up your regimen and where you might get in trouble along the way. Right after you take a moment to congratulate yourself on how far you've come, ask yourself, *Have I noticed that the more I move, the less I crave unhealthy foods?* If you've noticed that switch, that's fantastic! That means your brain is getting its feel-good hormone dopamine from movement rather than sweets and bad foods. There's no turning back now—you're on the wagon for good.

GOOD SORE VERSUS BAD SORE

If you've ever had an epic workout, especially if you haven't worked out in a couple of weeks or years, you are familiar with DOMS (delayed-onset muscle soreness). DOMS happens when you repetitively overexert a muscle group. You feel great immediately after the workout, and maybe for the rest of the day. Then you wake up the next morning and can barely lift your arms or walk upstairs. DOMS is an inflammatory response where you tore muscle cells so they can regenerate stronger and bigger. Sadly, stretching does not prevent delayed-onset muscle soreness. DOMS just happens, and you have to work through it. Ice doesn't help either, while we're debunking training myths. Despite every pro athlete owning a cryotank these days, there is no data on the effectiveness of cold therapy either (still, if you feel better, go for it). Taking a little ibuprofen helps you recover a bit faster. Many folks mistakenly attribute muscle soreness to excess lactic acid produced when the body works hard and has to get supermetabolic. Many fitness buffs do recovery workouts, stretch, and cross-train specifically to reduce lactic acid levels. But lactic acid buildup is not actually why you get sore. Your innards are fine with high levels of acid—the acid in the stomach is much higher than the acid your muscles produce. The acid in your kidneys and urine is also pretty high, and you don't pee fire (unless you do, then see your urologist STAT). The truth is, reducing lactic acid levels won't make DOMS go away. Time, reducing exercise intensity for a couple of days, and good sleep will assuage the DOMS.

THE SCIENCE (OR LACK THEREOF) BEHIND INFRARED SAUNAS

Infrared saunas are all the rage. The claims of infrared sauna are outstanding: better sleep, better exercise recovery, better skin, de-stressing (I want in!). It's true you get 25 to 45 minutes of relaxation during the sauna, perhaps some time to meditate, which will relieve your stress. Any high-heat environment will raise your heart rate and cause you to break a sweat, and that may make you more metabolic and burn fat. But a regular sauna does that as well. Another claim is that infrared saunas detoxify your body by causing you to sweat out more toxins than a traditional sauna. Yes, infrared saunas are cooler so you can safely stay in longer and sweat longer—but do toxins really travel with sweat? Sweat releases sodium and chloride and the tiniest bit of heavy metals like lead. Your kidneys and liver detox you. If you're sweating out toxins, that means you're in kidney and or liver failure and your sweat is trying to compensate. So there isn't much science behind infrared saunas. Bottom line: there's nothing wrong with infrared saunas, and if you think it feels good, do it.

Ice, Ice Maybe

If you live in a big city, I'm sure you've seen ads for storefronts where you can dunk yourself in an ice bath. Why? Maybe you think it reduces inflammation and speeds recovery. You've seen pitchers in the dugout with an ice pack wrapped around their throwing arm after they pitched six solid innings. Looks cool, maybe feels good, but does it help? Not really. Orthopedic surgeons have studied icing for 50 years and have yet to show good data that it does much of anything except inhibit wound healing. When you apply ice to a body part, the blood vessels contract—it's a physiologic response to shunt blood away from cold areas to preserve core temperature and keep you alive. But to heal a body part, you need good blood flow to carry nourishment to the injured area. Placing an ice pack doesn't help healing, because it slows blood flow, but it can make you feel better. Why? Ice numbs the area, so your pain diminishes. So a little ice is good for immediate pain relief and will reduce swelling—but you want a little swelling because that's your body trying to heal itself.

STRETCHING HELPS

Five minutes of stretching gets blood flow to muscles and goes a long way toward preventing injury, especially for those new to vigorous exercise. Stretching also improves range-of-motion performance in activities like tennis, basketball, or other dynamic exercises. Here are some quick and easy stretches:

Stretching

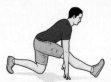

Half Split
Hold for 30 to 60 seconds each leg, repeat 2 to 5 times

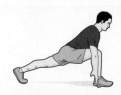

Runner's Lunge Stretch
Hold for 45 to 60 seconds each side, repeat 2 to 5 times

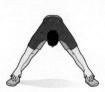

Wide-Stance Toe Touch
Hold 30 seconds, repeat 3 to 5 times

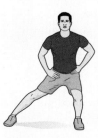

Adductor Stretch
Gently lean until you feel a good tug in your inner thigh, rock up and down for 5 seconds, switch legs

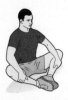

Seated Adductor Stretch
Place elbows on knees. Hold position for 5 to 10 seconds, repeat until inner thigh feels relaxed

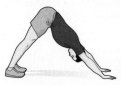

Calf Stretch (Downward Dog)
With hands and feet (as flat as you can) on the floor, press hips back and up, and hold for 5 to 10 seconds, repeat 2 to 3 times

Yoga Is for Everyone

Technology has made yoga accessible for almost everyone. You don't need a studio or a personal instructor. You can find guided classes online to get started. Yoga is a detailed, regimented form of stretching that encourages flexibility and can improve breathing, blood pressure, and athletic performance.

ROLL IT OUT

I love foam rolling—it is painful if you do it right but feels great when you finish. Yes, I like that hurt-so-good pain of deep stretching that foam rolling triggers. After a hard workout, using a foam roller and your body weight to rub down your muscles theoretically increases blood flow to the myofascia (the connective tissue of your muscle). Myofascial release helps recovery and restores muscle range of motion. But true myofascial release should be done by professionals, physical therapists, physical therapist assistants, and even properly trained massage therapists. Self-myofascial release through foam rolling has no data that supports its ability to improve recovery or performance. As with many do-it-yourself activities, you may achieve some benefit, but nothing replaces well-trained professionals to perform high-level treatment. But when I'm really in trouble, I see my physical therapist, who is a genius at getting me back to top athletic performance. See the next page for some stretches using a foam roller.

Roll It Out

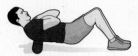

Upper Back Roll

With a foam roller under your upper back, arms crossed, raise your hips off of the ground, placing your weight onto the roller. Shift your weight to one side, rolling the upper to mid back. Alternate sides.

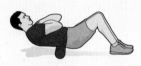

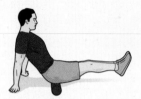

Lower Back Roll

Cross your arms in front of you, raise hips off the floor and lean back, keeping your weight on your lower back. Roll back and forward, keeping your weight off the spine and on the muscles. Repeat on the other side.

Hamstrings Roll

Place your hands to the side or behind you for support. Using your hands, lift hips off the floor and shift your weight on the foam roll to one leg (relax the hamstring of the leg you are stretching). Roll from below the hip to above the back of the knee. Repeat on opposite leg.

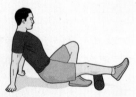

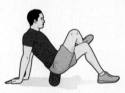

Calf Roll

Place hands at sides or just behind you, and press down to raise your hips off the floor, placing your weight against your calf muscle. Roll from below the knee to above the ankle. Repeat on opposite leg.

Glutes Roll

Sit with your butt on top of a foam roller. Bend your knees, and then cross one leg so that the ankle is over the knee. Shift your weight to the side of the crossed leg, rolling over your glutes until you feel tension. Repeat on opposite side.

GIVE YOUR BODY
A BOOST

The fitness landscape is flooded with supplements, none of which are FDA approved and all of which make some big promises. Most are bogus, but a few make some sense.

Creatine. This powder, usually added to a drink, is safe and can boost muscle mass, if you're trying to gain. Creatine is a muscle building block. How much you take depends on how much muscle you want to add. Typical dosing starts with a weeklong loading dose of 10 to 20 grams a day. After the first week, you can take anywhere from 2 grams a day for more aerobic performance improvement to 20 grams if you're trying to put on mass. If you have kidney disease or high blood pressure, check with your physician first. I always recommend increasing water intake while taking creatine—drink an extra liter or two of water a day to help metabolize the supplement. Creatine really works. There is data to support its use in both optimizing aerobic fitness for cardio-heavy sports and, at higher doses, improving muscle gain.

L-arginine/L-citrulline. These two closely related amino acids, or protein building blocks, are good for boosting nitric oxide in the muscles while exercising. Nitric oxide can improve blood flow and therefore may boost muscle energy. It will make you feel tingly and have itchy skin. Start slow with L-arginine and L-citrulline—like 500 milligrams a day—and work up. You can usually take up to 3,000 milligrams daily if you are getting a benefit. (By the way, citrulline can boost erections, so that's a bonus.) The difference between arginine and citrulline is timing. Your liver breaks arginine into nitric oxide just a few minutes after you ingest it, so it works fast but doesn't last long. Citrulline passes through the liver and into the bloodstream where, eventually, the kidney breaks it down into L-arginine. Citrulline therefore lasts longer—a slower burn—which is why I usually recommend it. These are safe supplements, and they occur in nature. Watermelon has an unbelievable level of citrulline (the Latin scientific name for watermelon is *Citrullus lanatus*).

Caffeine. Just like a simple cup of coffee, any form of caffeine is good for improving energy before a workout to help you push yourself harder. Thirty to 60 milligrams is a good dose to take an hour or so before a workout. I don't care how you get your caffeine: a cup of coffee or a natural energy drink. I like the tablets by Nuun that have balanced caffeine and electrolytes and none of the fake stuff.

B-complex vitamins. Do B vitamins improve energy in people who already have good nutritional habits? The scientific evidence is unclear. There is a whole industry of physicians and naturopaths who give B_{12} injections to boost energy. Data is weak that this does anything, but it's a pretty harmless practice. Vitamin B_6 is a critical part of hundreds of cellular reactions, from sugar to fat metabolism to nerve conduction. In developed countries, it's tough to be deficient in B_6 as the vitamin is found in meat, fruits, vegetables, and fish. But men with diabetes, obesity, kidney disease, and other chronic illnesses don't absorb B_6 as well. Taking a B-complex supplement isn't a bad idea to be sure, but don't expect it to change your life.

Electrolytes. You only need electrolytes—either your own concoction or in a sports drink—if you do hard-core sweating for at least 30 minutes. You know how I feel about sugary or sweetened drinks (see page 116), so seek out drinks that are just electrolytes and a little natural flavoring. There are electrolyte tabs you can dissolve in your water that work great and save money and reduce plastic bottle consumption.

⚠️ PROCEED WITH CAUTION
A Better Body through Steroids

Anabolic steroids, a form of high-dose synthetic testosterone, have long been used by men and women for simply looking jacked. Yes, they work. And yes, it is a shortcut. While you can certainly look shredded, lean, and defined *without* the help of anabolics, you probably can't look like Mr. Olympia, with massive muscles on top of muscles. You have to work out to get there. Hours and hours a day in the gym plus anabolic steroids will get you the superjacked look. Very skinny men that work out like crazy but can't gain mass will respond to anabolics. I understand the drive for these men to transform their bodies but they have to know the risks. The risks and side effects of using steroids are very real, but not everything you've heard is accurate. Will you get 'roid rage (no), will you grow breasts (maybe), will you get acne (yes), will your penis shrink (no), will your testicles shrink (yes), will you drop dead of a ruptured heart at 40? Probably not. Cardiovascular risks are minimal and overblown in the media. There was a lot of press around anabolic steroid abuse in the 1980s due to aggressive behaviors of pro wrestlers and other athletes who were juicing. The media tended to blame the anabolic steroids for the heart attacks

>>>

and wild behavior and not the cocaine these guys were simultaneously taking. However, the myth remains. I by no means advocate anabolic steroid use for anything other than medical indications, but I also don't want men perpetuating a myth.

The biochemical mechanism of steroids is pretty simple: anabolic steroids stimulate protein synthesis and, since muscles are protein, the muscle *really* grows. When properly prescribed, anabolic steroids serve a legitimate medical purpose—helping men who have wasting diseases like full-body burns, advanced cancers, and AIDS maintain muscle and weight. But like any drug, anabolic steroids can be dangerous if not well managed or are abused. For one, men who remain on these steroids for months and years at a time will blow out their pituitary glands to the point where they can never come off testosterone. When I see those men, they have the testosterone levels of a five-year-old boy, and they will need to take testosterone for the rest of their lives to feel normal. If you go the back-alley route, just know you may be taking horse testosterone from some offshore pharmacy with no standards. My best advice is to simply get back in the gym, put in the reps, and be proud of how great you look.

DON'T OVERDO IT

A lot of men who get really into fitness quickly realize there's a fine line between discipline and obsession. If you're that guy who has to do everything bigger, better, faster, stronger, and longer than everyone else, be careful. For most of us, it's tough to overexercise—we do too much, our body hurts, we stop. Too much too fast leads to burnout. Too much for too long can be worse. Some extreme athletes—ultramarathoners, for example—can ignore pain to the point where muscles break down (something called rhabdomyolysis) and their kidneys fail. Some guys become so committed to exercise they neglect relationships and other critical aspects of their life. Other men will turn to exercise as a way to cope with addiction, trading one compulsive behavior for another. That said, I'll take extreme fitness over alcoholism or drug addiction any day.

Chapter Cheat Sheet

☐ Don't make exercise complicated—just move a little more than you did yesterday.

☐ Hire a trainer if you're new to fitness.

☐ Get a heart rate monitor; target 80 percent of your max heart rate for at least 20 minutes a day.

☐ Stretching is your friend.

☐ Do it, but don't overdo it.

05

SEX

A Man's Guide to
the Good Stuff

Sex is fantastic. And it's also incredibly good for your health. **Sex brings you closer to your partner, which is good for de-stressing, and men who have more sex live longer and tend to be healthier and more active.** But which comes first: the sex or the healthy living? We know that the longer men and couples are sexually active, the longer they live. But you first have to be healthy enough to have sex. To have penetrative sex, a guy has to have a good erection (see page 168). Achieving and maintaining an erection is a physiological tour de force—a guy must have good heart and neurological function, good mental health, and solid testosterone levels. Bear in mind, each one of those faculties is also associated with longevity. So live it up and love it up!

The Perfect Sex Life Is a Myth

Too many men obsess over what is considered normal when it comes to how often they should be having sex. There is no *ab*normal, as long as you and your partner are happy. Have you always been less interested than what you *think* is typical for a guy? Maybe you spent time in the high school locker rooms listening to your teammates bragging about their conquests and you thought guys were having sex every day (that bragging guy was probably lying). Don't believe the hype. Statistics show that most men in long-term relationships have sex one or two times a week. But don't try to fit your sex life into a statistic. Some couples have sex daily, some once a month. Now if you and your partner are down to birthdays and leap years, that might be a different story, and it might be worth talking with a sex therapist.

MANAGING SEXPECTATIONS

It's not uncommon for two people in a relationship to have very different sex drives, and that can be tricky. Some men feel their libidos are in overdrive and their partners can't keep up. Some men feel they can't satisfy their partners with the amount of sex they want. We call it libido mismatch. It's crucial that you talk to each other. Maybe you need to adjust your routines or change what you do in the bedroom. Remember, too, that at least 70 percent of women will not orgasm with penile penetration alone. So if sex to you is *put it in, take it out, fall asleep*, your partner, especially a female partner, simply may not be getting much out of the experience.

The Mismatched Libido: Understand the Issue

Like all things sex, addressing a mismatched libido is complicated because sometimes the mismatch is physical, sometimes it's psychological, and sometimes it's situational. The first step is determining exactly what's going on by asking yourself a few questions.

1. Are you having a lot of solo sex?

This is common—men may have a strong desire for sexual release and masturbate to get the deed done without bothering their spouse. Some men don't want to invest the time into intimacy with a partner frequently and find it easier to rub one out than engage in coupling. This is less of a physiologic issue and more of a relationship and communication issue. If you find your lust for your partner lagging but not for your own kung fu grip, try backing off on the solo play and reengage your partner. You may be surprised by how much he or she is ready to engage right back at you.

2. Is the relationship otherwise okay?

If you and your partner are having trouble outside the bedroom, those difficulties will work their way into the bedroom. Don't drag this out. Have the conversation. Seek counseling if you can and are willing and rebuild the house before you rebuild the bedroom.

3. **Are you more stressed now than when you were first together?**

   If you are stressed, you may avoid intimacy instead of seeking intimacy as a stress reliever. But sex is a dopamine rush, a feel-good hormone boost that can, even temporarily, improve your response to stress. Relationships all start with a rush of dopamine—the newness of the partner, the excitement of the unknown. You put your previous life on hold to immerse yourself in his or her life. Then you settle down and realize you still have a previous life to balance, a job, friends, maybe kids, and, while all good things, they are stressful. Lean into your companion; a partner who is a keeper will be part of the solution.

4. **Is your testosterone low?**

   Low testosterone is the most common physiologic reason a guy has lost his libido. Tell your doc about your plummeting libido so you can have your testosterone levels checked.

KICK-START YOUR NEW SEX LIFE

Here are three tips for sparking a few flames.

Clean the House

Some very compelling studies have shown that men who perform housework enjoy more frequent sex. It makes a lot of sense, since your partner will be grateful and have fewer things on his or her to-do list. In heterosexual couples, multiple studies confirm frequency of sex correlates directly to how much of the household chores the man does. Whether you mow the lawn, take out the trash, or fold the laundry, your partner will reward you with more loving.

Schedule Sex

You're busy, your partner is busy, you don't have *time* for sex—I hear it all the time. But you've created routine in other areas of your life: mac and cheese Monday, taco Tuesday—why not hump day Wednesday? A lot of couples find that penciling in time for intimacy works wonders. We all think sex should be spontaneous and free, the way it was when our relationship just started. And it should be. But once you've built the foundation of a strong relationship, you may find less time to spark the sexual fire. Scheduling sex in between spontaneous rolls in the hay is a great way to show each other how important intimacy is to each of you. Make up a calendar code entry you both will recognize.

Communicate

Communicating with your partner is an amazing libido boost. The best time to talk about sex is outside of the bedroom. Keep a dialogue open with your partner to stoke the fires. Maybe you're interested in trying a new sex position—talk about it over dinner (assuming it's just the two of you). It turns out most people have sex fantasies that they don't often bring up with their partners. But do not suggest a new technique in the throes of passion—always let that passion go its own way, and next time you're thinking about sex, let your guy or gal know what's on your mind. Then the next time you're in bed, remind your partner about what you talked about.

PROCEED WITH CAUTION

Porn

Porn isn't what it used to be. As men now have millions of hours of porn video sitting in their pockets at any given time, porn is actually having a negative influence on men's sex lives. I'm seeing and hearing of more and more men who find it easier to ejaculate watching porn than while having sex with their partner. With such easy access to pornography, and from such a young age, many men spend more time with themselves than their partners, reaching a point where their penises are actually somewhat desensitized. For one, no orifice can provide the wall tension of a man's own hand, so if a guy spends more time masturbating than penetrating, the penis desensitizes and it takes more friction and more thrusting to get off (maybe even an impossible amount). Then there's the psychology component, in which men are drawn to the idea of getting off without having to invest in another person's pleasure. That's not only a mistake, it's a relationship problem. Believe it or not, there is a growing movement of men who are abstaining from masturbation to resensitize themselves. This is called the "nofap" movement—*fap*, repeated over and over, *fapfapfapfap*, refers to the sound of hand stroking penis. No lie. When I come across this in my practice, I rely on sex therapists to counsel these men and couples to establish more intimacy and less alone time.

The Orgasm, Explained

If you add up all men who orgasm too quickly, have trouble orgasming, or can't finish at all, it's a big slice of the male population. Thankfully, there are several solutions—technique, lifestyle, and often medication.

LIVE RIGHT, FINISH STRONG

Once again, eating right, moving more, and sleeping better will have a huge effect on your orgasms. If you're lean, in great shape, and sleeping perfectly, you'll experience better, stronger erections; the harder the penis, the more the nerve fibers are stretched. Sometimes guys don't realize that their erections are not 100 percent if they're still good enough for penetration. Meanwhile, the heavier you are, the less your penis shows, so fewer nerve fibers bring a pleasing feedback sensation to your brain. When you lose weight, your belly recedes and your penis has better exposure. **The take-home here is, strengthen your erections first, then let's see how we make the orgasms better and more frequent.**

There was a small study years ago where they gave men over age 65 with delayed or absent orgasms and normal erections a daily 5 milligram dose of tadalafil (Cialis), an erectile dysfunction drug. Scientists found that men were statistically more likely to orgasm on that drug. What that tells me is, those guys probably didn't have perfect erections. The tadalafil gave them a harder erection and that improved nerve conduction and their orgasms.

THE EJACULATION IMPULSE

Ejaculation is a neurologic and hormonal phenomenon. It's basically a reflex similar to when your doctor hits your knee with that rubber hammer. In the same way that some kick soft and some kick hard, men have varying degrees of sensitivity to ejaculation. There's a nerve at the tip of the penis, on the bottom side, right where your pee hole ends (the frenulum), that causes ejaculation once stimulated enough. Whereas some guys have a hair trigger and go off fast, other guys have a delayed trigger and it takes them longer to finish. Testosterone and a bunch of other hormones influence ejaculation intensity and time as well. The sensitivity in the frenulum can also be dialed too far up or down, leading to issues with premature ejaculation or delayed ejaculation.

Premature Ejaculation Is Misunderstood

I've had men tell me that their ejaculation dysfunction has ended what they thought were great relationships. Men have told me they are afraid to date because they were embarrassed by their loss of control and were self-conscious that they wouldn't stack up to the other lovers their partner has had in the past. And then there's the porn industry that shows men lasting forever without ejaculating. All of this can crush a man's ego. In counseling men who struggle with premature ejaculation (PE), I like to start by telling them what *won't* help before I talk about what will. I do this because too many men get the advice that PE is in their head and a behavioral thing. You cannot think this away. Contrary to what many men believe, PE is a physiological event, not psychological. Certainly, men with PE will have psychological components—it's distressing! But realize there are successful treatments, medical and psychological, so you don't have to live like this.

A man can actually train to delay his ejaculation, but it takes a willing partner and a lot of practice. We know that having intercourse more frequently increases ejaculation time, but that is usually not quite enough to solve the problem. If medical treatment is necessary, it's worth noting there are no FDA-approved medications for premature ejaculation. But there are drugs prescribed off-label that can help (an off-label drug is a drug approved by the FDA for other uses that doctors repurpose for a different illness).

Many men will say they orgasm quickly the first time, then, 20 minutes later, they're hard again and ready to go at it for longer. Problem is, your partner may be asleep by then. So here are some common methods for treating premature ejaculation.

How to Slow Things Down: Home Remedies

Start-stop. Sex therapists describe a start-stop technique, where a man thrusts for a bit and stops, then restarts. This may work for some couples, but it can be a source of frustration for the partner and his or her libido. They could be getting in a great rhythm, then their man suddenly stops. And for many men, milliseconds before they stop, they've already reached the point of no return and let loose.

The pinch. An offshoot of this technique is to pull out entirely and pinch the head of the penis hard enough to hurt. The thought is that this resets the ejaculatory reflex. Truthfully, I've never met a man who told me that it works, though it could be that the pinch is effective and that's why they don't seek my treatment. Either way, this technique is harmless and worth a try before you make an appointment with a doctor or therapist.

Edging. Dating back to ancient sex manuals like the Kama Sutra, edging occurs when a guy stimulates to the point of orgasm and stops for a long time—like minutes, hours, or even days. The idea is that when he finally orgasms, it will take longer to get there and be more intense. It's harmless and worth a try. Problem is, for men with a serious premature ejaculation issue, the nerve reflex is just too strong and they release before they get a chance to edge. This is just a marathon start-stop.

Edging is a common technique for those who are into tantric sex, the ancient practice of intercourse without orgasming every time. Tantric sex heightens intimacy and connection since the lovemaking lasts longer than the usual 5 to 20 minutes and allows for more full-body exploration. Then, after a few sessions of tantric sex, a man completes the act and ejaculates—the orgasm is supposedly much more intense. Again, edging is in no way dangerous, though it is essentially self-induced blue balls and may cause a dull ache in the testicles after a trip to the edge.

Numbing cream. Topical numbing creams and sprays work great for premature ejaculation, and I recommend these to all my patients prior to trying prescription drugs. Essentially, you smear or spray a numbing agent like lidocaine on the head of your penis and let it soak in for about 15 minutes. Unless you're wearing a condom, it might be a good idea to wash it off before penetration, so you don't inadvertently also numb your partner. Some of the better formulations fully absorb. There are a lot of brands; Promescent leads the market because their products fully absorb to minimize transference to your partner, and they have invested the most research into the field of transdermal delivery mechanisms. You can get them online or at many drugstores and pharmacies. These creams work way better than the behavioral techniques I just mentioned.

Don't be discouraged if you can't solve your rapid orgasm time at home. There are a few good medical solutions that your urologist can prescribe to delay your finish time.

How to Slow Things Down: Medical Remedies

<u>Antidepressant medications.</u> A common off-label treatment for PE, antidepressants slow ejaculation by blocking the hormone serotonin. They work best if taken daily, but they do have side effects, especially if you're not depressed, that commonly include dry mouth, drowsiness, restlessness, and occasionally anxiety. They may also cause some GI issues like nausea and constipation. But overall, these are very well-tolerated medications that can change a guy's (and his partner's) life.

<u>Tramadol.</u> The other big off-label drug is tramadol (also sold as Ultram), a painkiller related to narcotics. There are very few side effects, but there is a concern you may develop a dependency. I've prescribed tramadol for premature ejaculation because it works, but I do have to counsel my patients about its off-label use. You don't have to take it every day, just a half hour before sex to delay ejaculation.

WHAT IF YOU CAN'T REACH THE FINISH LINE?

Delayed ejaculation—anorgasmia or anejaculation—is when it takes too long for a man to orgasm or he can't finish at all. We don't have good statistics on how many men suffer from anorgasmia, but in my practice, it's a common problem. It gets progressively worse with age and mostly happens in older men. I see a spike in delayed ejaculation in men over 60, and it worsens the older men get. Physiologically, it's pretty much the opposite of premature ejaculation: instead of being too sensitive, the nerves that fire during orgasm are blunted. I have to say, this is one of the most frustrating conditions to deal with as we simply don't have any mainstream therapies. It can be devastating to men. Their partners tend to take it personally. I will also say, you have to have realistic expectations. As we age, we lose a few steps—we don't run as fast, we don't see as well, we don't lift as much. So it stands to reason that we don't orgasm as well.

While there are a few things you can try yourself, medical treatment may be a better option. There are five hormones that need to be at optimal levels to orgasm and ejaculate: testosterone, serotonin, dopamine, prolactin, and oxytocin. Dopamine is the feel-good hormone, and getting those levels up pharmacologically is tough. Of those hormones, we can only clinically test prolactin and testosterone—the rest have no established reference ranges. Testosterone is easy. If your T levels are low, you may improve orgasm by boosting testosterone through replacement therapy (more on that in the testosterone section on page 39). Prolactin levels should be under 16 nanograms per milliliter in an adult male. Over that number suggests prolactin could impair orgasmic response. If prolactin levels are even higher, it may mean your pituitary gland is oversecreting the hormone because you have a noncancerous tumor called a prolactinoma. If your prolactin level is above 20, your physician may order a pituitary scan.

As with drugs used to treat premature ejaculation, there are no FDA-approved medications specifically for delayed ejaculation. There are, however, some off-label drugs that can work. Here are a few options for treating DE if it has become an issue.

Delayed Ejaculation: Home Remedies

Good vibes. The ejaculatory trigger nerve center, known as the frenulum, is on the bottom of the penis, just where the tip meets the shaft. If you apply a vibrating stimulus to this area, you can trigger the response. There are lots of vibrating adult sex aids for men—I'll leave that up to you and your internet search engine to find one that works for you and your partner(s).

Kegel reps, not just for women. Kegel exercises engage the ejaculatory muscles, although they were developed to help women regain urinary control after childbirth. The next time you urinate, stop your flow midstream and concentrate on the action; hold for just a few seconds, then finish urinating. That's a Kegel (once you get that muscle down, stop doing it when you pee, as it feels pretty weird). A good routine is to hold for a five-second count, relax, and repeat three to five times, around ten times a day. You can do Kegels just about anywhere—red-light Kegels are all the rage here in Los Angeles since we spend so much time in traffic.

DIEGO, 33

It Was All in His Head

Diego is a 33-year-old male who came to me for an infertility evaluation. He and his wife had been trying to conceive for over a year with no luck. He mentioned to me that one problem, in addition to his fatigue, stress, loss of libido, and poor erections, was he couldn't ejaculate most of the time. His wife took it personally, even felt Diego didn't want to have a kid. Diego certainly had multiple symptoms of low testosterone, but the inability to ejaculate suggested his prolactin levels were high. His blood work showed he had severely low testosterone but also a dramatically high prolactin level. This prompted me to order an MRI of his pituitary gland that revealed a pituitary tumor. While no one wants to hear he has a tumor, Diego was relieved when I let him know medication would shrink the tumor and he would likely recover his testosterone and ejaculatory function. Sure enough, after two months of taking the drug cabergoline to lower his prolactin, his erections, testosterone, and ejaculation improved, and the couple conceived.

Supplements. No supplements will help make you orgasm sooner, though supplements that improve nitric oxide flow to the penis may help. L-arginine and L-citrulline (the first is shorter acting than the second) have been shown to increase penile engorgement and may help orgasm, but no studies involving these supplements have specifically addressed orgasmic dysfunction. You can take up to 3,000 milligrams a day of arginine or citrulline, split into a morning and an evening dose. Most men will feel a little energy boost, a little skin tingle as it dilates the skin blood vessels also.

Just as you can't always cure premature orgasm at home, you may find you need medical help to diagnose and treat delayed orgasm as well. Your urologist may have some medical therapies that could work.

Delayed Ejaculation: Medical Remedies

Cabergoline. This is effective in reducing high prolactin levels, which can be caused by growths on the pituitary gland. Cabergoline is safe, has very few side effects, and can improve orgasm in men with normal prolactin levels. There are rare reports of men with compulsive behaviors like gambling or other addictions becoming more compulsive on the drug, but this is uncommon and not really proven. All the same, if you have a history of compulsive behavior, tell your doctor before he or she prescribes you cabergoline.

Oxytocin. The "cuddle hormone" releases at the point of orgasm in men *and* women, and boosting levels during sex can sometimes help stimulate an orgasm. Usually, oxytocin comes as a nasal spray men whiff at the beginning, or even during, intercourse, as it is very short acting (like eight minutes). Some of my patients have had great success and others have seen no results, but I haven't had anyone complain about side effects. Therefore, I put this in the "can't hurt, might help" category.

SEX AND GETTING STONED

Men who smoke weed daily have a tougher time reaching orgasm. However, a little weed could be good for guys prone to premature ejaculation. That said, we know that frequent marijuana use may decrease sperm function and also lower testosterone levels. On a high note, a recent study out of Stanford showed that couples who smoke weed frequently wanted to have *more* sex than sober counterparts. But as with alcohol, if you're trying to initiate a pregnancy and it's not happening, cut out the weed to be safe. If you suffer from anxiety (sexual anxieties, in particular), you may find that moderate weed usage helps with that. Just don't gain too much weight from the weed munchies.

The Importance of a Good Erection

Show me a man with a normal erection, and I'll show you a healthy man with a healthy heart. Men who develop erectile dysfunction in their 40s are twice as likely to experience a cardiovascular problem in the next 10 years as men with normal erections. This is not to scare you but rather an admonition to not only improve your erections, but also your heart health.

"MORNING WOOD" IS GOOD

Morning erections are your body's way of saying *all systems go*. If you get regular morning erections, it means you have good cardiovascular health, good testosterone levels, you're getting enough sleep, and you have good blood flow to the penis. A healthy man might get morning wood, even if he is not able to get an erection when he's awake. Erectile dysfunction is often tied to anxiety. When a man is in deep REM sleep, his body and brain are essentially shut off and his pituitary gland sends a signal to the testicles to make more testosterone. Indeed, T levels are highest in the early morning in healthy men under age 50. When a man is sleeping soundly, his stress hormones are low.

> **A CALL TO ACTION** If you ever stop getting morning erections, it's time to see your doctor. Maybe it's as simple as weight gain or not getting enough

sleep. But it is a sign that the wheels have come off somewhere along the road and it's time to do something about it.

ERECTIONS AT 80 YEARS OLD

You're never too old to get an erection and have intercourse. Sure, it's normal for most men to have less-frequent intercourse the older they get, but this isn't universal, and what is normal for one man may be abnormal for another. When I see a man in his 60s with erectile dysfunction and he tells me maybe he's just too old to have sex, it saddens me. I ask him if he's too old to read or is he okay wearing reading glasses, since the older we get, the more we need glasses. Fact is, I see men in their 80s and 90s who enjoy a very active sex life with their partners. There are some studies that show what is normal by decade for frequency of sex, but I don't care much about those guidelines—I care about what a man wants. If he and his partner feel great having sex every day or every week or once a month, it's all good.

MARTY, 85

Going Strong in the Golden Years

Marty is a healthy 85-year-old man I've seen for years for mild erectile dysfunction. He keeps in great shape, swims in the Santa Monica Bay three to five days a week, and has been taking 100 milligrams of Viagra, the maximum dose, for more than ten years with great results. Until one day, it stopped working. His girlfriend wasn't too stressed, as they still had great intimacy together, just not penetrative sex. But he was bothered—he didn't think being 85 was an excuse for why his erections weren't working. And he was right. I quickly ruled out many medical reasons for his worsening ED, from heart failure to diabetes—all normal. I did check his testosterone again, as it was normal five years earlier when he was doing great. Sure enough, his T levels had dropped well below normal range. After starting him on testosterone therapy, Marty got a great response again to Viagra and was back to his raging 85-year-old erection.

ERECTILE DYSFUNCTION, DEMYSTIFIED

Anytime a man is unable to achieve an erection good enough for penetration, and sustain it long enough to orgasm, he has ED. An erection requires four systems to be firing on all cylinders: blood flow to the penis; nerves telling the muscles in the penis to relax and allow that blood to flow; hormones, like testosterone and nitric oxide, stimulating the sexual thoughts and triggering the nerves to fire; and, perhaps the most complex of all, being "in the mood." Before the invention of Viagra, doctors blamed ED on that last factor 90 percent of the time, saying it was psychological, not physiological.

Post-Viagra, it's the other way around. But I say those perspectives are both wrong, because if you take a totally normal guy and put him in a situation where he can't get an erection, that's going to cause some psychological damage. And that's why I always treat men for both.

SEE A DOCTOR IMMEDIATELY IF . . .

You Develop Erectile Dysfunction Before Age 50

If you're 40 and you have ED, you need to see your physician to evaluate whether you have any heart problems. It may be nothing, but you should at least get your blood pressure and cholesterol checked and let your doctor know if you have a family history of heart disease and early death. As I mentioned earlier (and this is worth repeating), **men who develop ED before age 50 have a higher risk of cardiovascular disease and of having a heart attack within ten years of their ED diagnosis**. This shouldn't scare you—it should motivate you.

Erectile Dysfunction: Things You Can Try Before You See Your Doc

Thankfully, ED is something men have more control over than they think, and it does not always require medical treatment. My primary question is whether the problem is situational or chronic. Before you even visit the doctor, ask yourself a few questions (they're the same ones I'm going to ask you): *Do you wake up most mornings with an erection? Do you get normal erections when you have sex while on vacation? Do you get an erection when you masturbate?*

If the answer is yes to any of the above, you are likely in good shape, *medically*. Very often, there is an anxiety component to getting an erection with a partner, and this usually calls for less-invasive therapy. Thus, these home remedies for addressing the psychological or emotional component are often effective:

Relax. I see so many guys in my clinic who are young, often under 40, even, and stressed beyond belief. That stress carries into the bedroom. He starts getting anxious about whether he'll get an erection or not, and his adrenaline levels spike. This fight-or-flight hormone shunts blood away from the penis, pumping it all into the heart and skeletal muscles. That takes all the blood flow from the penis and leaves him limp at the wrong time. This can be a vicious cycle. For some men, just knowing this is what is happening helps. But it's also good to remember that foreplay isn't just for women— the more time a man spends relaxing and initiating intimacy, the more likely the erection will come back to life.

Go on vacation. Perhaps you don't know the answer to the vacation sex question above—well, now is the time to find out. Vacation sex is awesome. You and your partner are relaxed, rested, have a room to yourself (I hope), and all of this exhilarates a man, increases libido, and thus, often increases erectile strength and frequency.

Schedule sex. Even if the vacation sex is fantastic, it can often go right back to less than fantastic once you return to your stressful routines—work, yard work, kids' soccer games. The best thing for you and your partner to do here is carve out time to improve sex at home. Some couples find scheduling sex helps them commit. Don't force it, though. Some partners may feel pressured that it's another chore on the to-do list. The best thing is to come up with the plan outside of the bedroom and see if it resonates with your partner.

Press pause on the porn. This is especially important if you are getting erections when you're by yourself but not with your partner. I see this more and more frequently.

Try the right natural supplement. Many natural remedies are mere myths: fenugreek, horny goat weed, deer and elk antler extract are all a waste of money. There are, however, a couple of natural supplements that have shown promise to treat ED and might be worth a try:

- **L-citrulline.** This improves nitric oxide levels, which act similar to Viagra in relaxing smooth muscle in the penis to allow more blood flow. L-citrulline is a naturally occurring amino acid found in high concentrations in watermelon. It's not only good for erections but for gains at the gym. Many workout drinks contain arginine or citrulline to add a little extra pump to a workout. Arginine and citrulline are essentially the same, but arginine is cleared in the liver, so it is metabolized and burned up much faster than citrulline, which is cleared by the kidney. Some supplements combine arginine, for a quick-acting nitric oxide boost, and citrulline, for the delayed response. For erectile dysfunction, you want the slow burn of citrulline—typically around 1,500 to 3,000 milligrams a day.

- **Korean ginseng.** Most studies show dosages up to 900 milligrams, three times a day, can improve erections. But that is a lot of capsules and can get pretty expensive.

- **Beetroot extract and ginger.** These supplements to improve blood flow are pretty hot these days. Beetroot is a natural source of nitric oxide, which stimulates relaxation of the penile muscles to allow more blood flow in and harder erections. There is a very well-studied, scientifically scrutinized supplement called Revactin, which is a proprietary blend of ginger and other nitric oxide supplements that has very good randomized controlled data.

- **Maca.** There is a very weak signal that maca, a standard to any male virility supplement, may have a small effect on erections. Some men swear by maca—it's the root of a plant that grows at altitude in the Andes mountains and has been harvested for centuries by the Incas as a natural fertility and erection booster. There are really no side effects, and therefore I don't discourage taking it.

Erectile Dysfunction: Medical Remedies

Pills. ED drugs relax smooth muscle to allow more blood to flow into the penis. These pills—drugs like sildenafil, tadalafil, and avanafil, found in medications like Viagra, Cialis, and Stendra, respectively—have been around for over 20 years now and are safe for almost all men (men taking nitroglycerin for severe heart disease need to get cleared by their cardiologist). While these drugs used to be very expensive and rarely covered by insurance, that's changed. Sildenafil and tadalafil, for example, are generic, and many pharmacies sell these medications for less than a dollar a pill. In my practice, my goal is to get men off these medications after a few months and help them restore normal sexual function with lifestyle modification. But if a man needs a pill, this is a solid long-term—and usually safe—option. I generally start men on a low daily dose of the medications, 5 milligrams a day for tadalafil or 20 milligrams a day for sildenafil, which tends to minimize the side effects and allows men to be more spontaneous in intercourse. Tadalafil has a longer length of action so this is usually my first go-to. Side effects are minimal for most men—mild headache, stuffy nose, mild heartburn, or muscle ache. For some, however, the side effects are miserable and therefore these pills aren't a good choice for them.

Pokes. Intracavernosal injections (ICIs) have been around for nearly 40 years, and they work really well for treating ED. But you have to be willing to stick a needle in your penis and give yourself—or have your partner give you—an injection to stoke an erection. It's the same size needle and amount of medicine as you'd get with a flu shot, like an eyedropper full of medicine, and most men barely feel the needle. But the erection itself can be raging, even too much of a good thing. Dosing the amount of medicine is critical: too little and you won't get an erection, too much and the erection doesn't go away and can even damage the penis. Partners usually like the injection because the erection is superrigid, but it can be a bit much for the patient.

Procedures. The gold-standard ED procedure remains the penile implant, which is great for men who can't achieve erections through more conservative therapies. The penile implant comes in two main forms: a semirigid rod or an inflatable implant filled with salt water. Both are inserted during a surgical procedure that lasts about an hour. I equate the penile implant with a joint replacement. When your knee starts to go, your physician prescribes a pill like ibuprofen. When that stops working, you move on to injections into the joint. When those fail, you get a knee replacement. A penile implant will give you satisfying, long-lasting erections that most closely simulate what your erection felt like before you had ED. Pick out an experienced surgeon for this procedure, as the complications can be rough. If the implant develops an infection, it has to be removed, which leads to scar tissue, making a second surgery even more difficult. Penile implant surgeries are some of the most satisfying surgeries I perform. To restore lost intimacy to men and their partners motivates me.

A Moment to Honor the Little Blue Pill

It's been over 20 years since Viagra (sildenafil) came to market and revolutionized men's health. I argue that Viagra actually *created* the field of men's health. A man doesn't typically go to the doctor for routine checkups. But if his penis stops working and he knows a doctor can write a prescription to jump-start it, he'll make an appointment immediately. Before we had a national conversation about ED, men would go decades without seeing a physician—decades full of bad decisions like overeating, overdrinking, smoking, and not knowing they were developing chronic illnesses like diabetes or high blood pressure. All these medical problems cause erectile dysfunction and, therefore, are targets for a physician to manage and improve. It was the little blue pill that started the conversation that has led to millions of men establishing care with a physician. Men now have a good reason for seeing doctors and getting checked up and checked out.

Blood Pressure Meds Cause ED

There's a common myth that blood pressure medication causes erectile dysfunction. Here's the deal: *high blood pressure* (HBP) itself causes erectile dysfunction. The longer you have high blood pressure, the worse off your penis will be—and your eyes, kidneys, brain, heart, and the rest of your vital organs. Anything you do to lower your blood pressure *improves* your ED. It's true that some high blood pressure meds can make erections weaker (beta-blockers, in particular), but these drugs save lives. As a doctor that treats ED, I typically leave your blood pressure medication alone and figure out a treatment strategy that complements their action. Since HBP is such an important cause of premature death and organ failure in men, I want to keep both your blood pressure and your penis happy. So I advise guys to stay on their blood pressure medication, but I also push the idea of developing better lifestyle habits. If you take medications for HBP, let's first see what happens when you get on a good weight-loss program, increase exercise, and consistently get at least six hours of sleep a night. Maybe that will let you stop taking your HBP medication.

ED TREATMENTS TO AVOID

As you can imagine, the ED industry is big bucks and there are lots of unscrupulous people. Yes, even physicians will try to sell you on something that doesn't work. Mostly, these therapies are not harmful, and you're only losing money. However, some can be dangerous, so be careful if you're seeking ED treatments from somewhere other than a reputable urologist.

Hi-Tech Remedies

There are a few new technologies and procedures to treat ED, but newer doesn't necessarily mean better. Among them is low-intensity shockwave therapy (LISWT) and stem cell or platelet-rich plasma injections into the penis. Neither is FDA approved or regulated, and while there are some randomized clinical trials showing some efficacy for LISWT, there's not much evidence out there backing injections. Plus, these are all expensive therapies, not covered by insurance. I recommend at least seeing a good urologist and pinning him or her down on outcomes and expectations before going this route. LISWT is first line therapy in Europe, but we just don't have the robust clinical trials to strongly recommend this technology.

Over-the-Counter Erection Meds

Step up to the cash register at any truck stop, convenience store, or gas station and you will see all sorts of sexual enhancement pills. Guys spend billions of dollars on mostly worthless supplements every year. Please don't. The FDA does not approve or regulate these supplements so anyone can put anything they want in a bottle and sell it. They all have catchy names and promise increasing your penis size, keeping you hard for *hours,* and whatever other lies they'll tell to sell. Fact is, these supplements can be anything from useless and harmless to effective but dangerous and even lethal. Avoid these things and spend your money on medications that work.

SEE A DOCTOR IMMEDIATELY IF . . .
You Have an Erection Injury

Normally, anything that makes a man's penis bigger should be a good thing, right? Not when it comes to *eggplant penis*. Imagine having vigorous, awesome sex and then, bam! You slam your erect penis into the pubic bone of your partner. You hear a sickening pop and your erect penis goes immediately flaccid. Minutes later, you see bruising and your penis swells and turns purple. You're sure you just broke your penis. But the penis isn't actually a bone; this is a rupture—the tough membrane that keeps your erection intact tore when the penis slammed into a hard structure. All the blood that is throbbing into the erection shoots out of the ruptured membrane and your penis looks like an eggplant. This is a surgical emergency: if you don't get it fixed soon, you have a 50 percent chance of erectile dysfunction. The surgical fix is to sew the ruptured membrane back together, so the penis doesn't explode every time you get an erection. How does one prevent corporal rupture? Coordination, my friend. Interestingly, most penile fractures occur when men—and possibly their partners—have put back a few too many drinks and lose their carnal rhythm.

THE CONSTRICTION TRADITION

One potential workaround for ED—specifically, for men who have trouble maintaining an erection—is the use of a penile occlusive band, a.k.a. a cock ring. Sometimes used as a sex toy (see page 52), cock rings can be rolled or cinched onto the base of the penis, or around the base of the penis and scrotum, as a way of engorging it with blood. To get an erection, the penis's arteries pump blood under high pressure until the erection is firm. Veins then slowly trickle blood out to keep a healthy flow of oxygenated blood. Some men have too much blood leak out during an erection (a condition called venous leak). A cock ring compresses the veins and keeps the penis harder during sex. Just remember, the oxygenated blood has to keep flowing in order to keep the penile tissue alive, so if you're choking off the inflow for too long, you may injure your penis permanently.

The Age of ED Drug Delivery

Online direct-to-consumer pharmacies are on the rise, many of which sell ED pills. All it requires is a quick online interview with a physician, who will send you a prescription after asking some very basic health questions. The advantages are you don't need to see a doctor in person and it's little to no wait for an appointment. If you're a young man, beware: you probably don't want to be taking ED pills for the rest of your life—especially if your physician finds something he or she can reverse. And that's the biggest downside, as you don't get a physical exam or blood work that may identify a more serious health condition. My research team recently published an article showing that not getting a comprehensive medical evaluation with a physical exam and blood work misses a lot of medical conditions that need attention. We looked at approximately 400 men under age 40 who came to my office because they were having trouble with their erections. Almost 40 percent of the time, I found a problem on these men's physical exams or in their blood work. Things like undiagnosed diabetes, high cholesterol, or low testosterone were common. Now if you can't wait for an office visit and really need to get a prescription, I think a reputable online pharmacy is fine, as long as you follow up in person with your doctor for a general checkup. But as with all things in men's health, if you simply eat better, move more, and sleep better, your erections should get better without logging in to a prescription service.

Chapter Cheat Sheet

☐ Erectile dysfunction isn't normal and can be a sign of other health concerns.

☐ Good nutrition, exercise, and sleep are natural ways to improve your erections.

☐ Great medical treatments exist to restore erection health in men.

☐ Ejaculation disorders are frustrating but usually treatable.

☐ The best way to improve your sex life is to communicate with your partner.

☐ Sex at any adult age is a sign of good health.

☐ There are some effective supplements for ED but don't wait too long to see your physician for more help.

06

FERTILITY

A Man's Guide to Procreation

Most heterosexual men spend their adolescence, twenties, and beyond trying to prevent impregnating someone. The fear is so ingrained for many guys that it may come as a surprise that many couples struggle to get pregnant. A lot has to go right for the sperm to find that egg and unravel the magic of pregnancy. For many couples, it's easy: penis in, and 10 months later, baby out. But fertility issues represent a large part of my practice. And they are on the rise. Maybe it's that many couples delay pregnancy to achieve higher professional status. Maybe it's due to the fact that men's sperm counts have declined over the decades. Researchers aren't sure if that is from environmental toxins or that men are less healthy than they were years ago—men are more obese, don't exercise as much, and probably stress more than previous generations. Better nutrition, exercise, and sleep all can improve your chances of initiating a pregnancy. Yep, stick to the principles and you'll be on track.

Sperm: The Swimmers

When it comes to good old-fashioned spontaneous pregnancy, *a lot* has to go right for one lucky sperm to get from a man's testicle all the way into a woman's reproductive tract. First, a man has to have an erection hard enough to penetrate the vagina. Next, the man has to be able to ejaculate the sperm as close to the cervix as possible for the sperm to start its journey up the female reproductive tract to find the egg. Typically, a man ejaculates over 40 million sperm with each orgasm. Thankfully, only one needs to go the distance. It sounds like better odds than it really is—the relative distance a sperm has to swim to find an egg is roughly the equivalent of a six-foot-tall man running from Los Angeles to San Francisco. And once that sperm reaches the egg, it's still not finished. That sperm then has to burrow into the egg wall—sperm don't actually swim; new microscopic video shows they burrow like drill bits—and unravel its DNA, hoping it lines up with the female DNA, so all chromosomes align and develop into an embryo. Every step of the way, there may be problems (many of which are on the male side). In this chapter, we're going to learn how to give those sperm the best chances of finding that egg and making a baby.

THE SEMEN ANALYSIS

The fundamental evaluation of a man's fertility is the semen analysis, in which a man provides a semen sample either by masturbating into a cup or with assistance of his partner in a locked room in my clinic (or he can bring a sample from home as long as it gets to my lab within 45 minutes). That sample then sits for a while to liquefy until my technologists analyze it. They're looking for four things: volume (how much liquid semen a man ejaculates); sperm counts, in which we use a standard formula to estimate the number of sperm in a sample (a fertile man ejaculates over 40 million sperm a shot); motility, or how many are moving and how fast they are moving (a man can have 40 million sperm but if none is moving, he's most likely infertile); and morphology, or the shape of the sperm, as sperm need to have pointy heads, dainty necks, and whippy tails to be morphologically normal. In a normal sperm sample, 4 percent of the sperm meet these strict criteria.

However, many physicians—even fertility specialists—probably don't know what a poor predictor the semen analysis is for pregnancy. Unfortunately, it's the best test we've got. When I counsel my male patients, I let them know that there is so much we *don't* know about fertility, and the semen analysis proves this uncertainty. Unless a man has zero sperm in his ejaculate, I can't say he's infertile. On the other hand, while I might be able to make your sperm counts look great, if you're not getting pregnant, I haven't helped you much. I don't want to be that doctor that tells a couple they'll never get pregnant with his low sperm counts. I've seen natural pregnancies in men with really poor sperm counts and seen couples struggle, despite great sperm counts.

Sperm and Semen Are Two Different Things

A lot of guys think sperm and semen are equivalent. Semen is the liquid portion of ejaculation, produced by the prostate gland and the seminal vesicles. Testicles produce sperm. The epididymis stores sperm. When a man ejaculates, sperm come up from the testicle and epididymis via the vas deferens and mix with semen coming from the prostate and seminal vesicles. The whole mixture comes together in the urethra (the same tube urine exits through). Semen is a viscous pudding that is filled with fructose, a sugar the sperm needs to move, and minerals like zinc that support sperm vitality and alkali to keep the pH of semen basic. The sperm needs a high pH because the vagina is naturally acidic to protect women from bacteria. If a sperm hits an acid environment, it dies, so the buffering of semen keeps the pH perfect for sperm to pass through the vagina on its way to its final destination.

A CALL TO ACTION I typically tell couples to try to conceive for 6 months, assuming they know how to track the wife's ovulation or are at least taking multiple shots on goal. If they haven't achieved pregnancy in 6 months, I recommend both man and woman get evaluated to optimize their fertility or identify any obvious barriers to conception.

Boosting Fertility

While a semen analysis is far from perfect in determining a man's fertility, it's the best screening tool we have. And if that test indicates an issue, it's time to try a few things to increase the little swimmers' odds. For me, a man's fertility status is a good indicator of overall health, which is why lifestyle changes are often so effective. A lot of recent research suggests that men with fertility troubles have higher rates of chronic diseases and cancer risk as they age. This isn't a scare tactic, but it is a good wake-up call for men to get their fertility status checked out. My research group recently published a paper showing that about 20 percent of men under age 40 with erectile dysfunction have abnormal sperm tests. As with most things in men's health, the eat-move-sleep triad can lead to optimal fertility. So, *before* pills or procedures, I start with a bit of preaching.

BOOSTING FERTILITY: HOME REMEDIES

Lose weight. Obesity is probably the most common reversible cause of male infertility. Being overweight decreases sperm counts *and* quality. Many obese men have low testosterone, and sperm need high levels of T in the testicle to function normally. Likewise, many obese men have high levels of estrogen, which decreases sperm production. Lastly, obese men often generate a lot more heat around their testicles, simply from the mass of their thighs and groin. Heavy guys tend to be more sedentary, which decreases the amount of time the testicles can dangle freely and cool naturally.

Stock up on sperm-boosting foods. Study after study demonstrates that eating high-quality whole foods improves fertility, and a few small dietary changes have dramatic effects. Leafy green vegetables, dark-colored fruits and berries (like blueberries), and tree nuts (like walnuts) have all been shown to improve sperm quality. Sperm are coated in poly-unsaturated fatty acids (PUFAs), and tree nuts—especially walnuts—are packed full of PUFAs. Fast and processed foods, on the other hand, are not great for sperm health—or for your overall health, for that matter. If it's not good for you, it's not good for your sperm.

Exercise. I've had a lot of men ask me if they should give up cycling because it kills sperm. The answer is a hard no. Sure, if you're cycling 100 miles a day, you may be impairing your sperm because the testicles are too hot and your testosterone levels drop when you're doing anything extreme (if you're pedaling your way down to 5 percent body fat, or cycling until your penis is numb, back off). But for the other 99.9 percent of men, cycling is one of the best exercises out there for weight loss, overall health, and thus, probably improving fertility. Any exercise you do—except maybe hot yoga (gotta keep the boys cool)—will improve your fertility.

Get a good night's sleep. Sleep deprivation *tanks* testosterone levels in men (see page 217 about getting sleep). The sperm production hormone comes from the pituitary gland near the brain. When you don't sleep, your pituitary gland doesn't sleep, and it stops making the sperm-signaling hormone.

Seek out sperm-boosting supplements. Thanks to so much research in fertility supplements, some high-quality fertility supplements are now available. There are also a lot of people trying to sell you stuff that they've never tested. As I've pointed out, the FDA does not regulate the supplement industry. If I wanted to sell you a gumdrop and tell you it is Dr. Mills's proven fertility booster, I could. The best supplement companies do research and publish their data in medical journals. One supplement brand that has spent a lot of money on high-level research is PROfertil. They provide pharmaceutical-grade supplements and have many randomized trials demonstrating a benefit to sperm quality. There are many competitors out there; I encourage you to research them and see what data they have before dropping the cash on supplements. You could save some money and buy the active ingredients separately as well. Selenium, coenzyme Q10, L-carnitine, folic acid, and vitamin C have all shown some improvements to sperm parameters in multiple randomized trials. The supplements I list above all have been through randomized controlled trials, the highest level of clinical evidence, that prove they work. Dosage varies depending on formulation, so I would leave it up to you to read the labels.

Here's my recommended sperm-boosting supplement daily regimen:

- Vitamin C: 500 mg a day
- Coenzyme Q10: 200 mg a day
- L-carnitine: 1,000 mg a day
- Folic acid: 400 mg a day
- Fish oil: 1,000 mg a day (this boosts ejaculate volume)

BOOSTING FERTILITY: WITH THE HELP OF SCIENCE

Only when lifestyle changes are not enough to boost a man's fertility do I turn to pills and procedures.

Pills. A lot of medications improve fertility, but one size does not fit all. To prescribe the correct medication to a man to boost his fertility, I'll need to know things like his hormone levels (particularly testosterone, estradiol, luteinizing hormone, follicle-stimulating hormone, and prolactin, which are all part of a standard fertility panel). These blood tests are not part of your primary doctor's normal healthy-man screening, so I check these at almost every new patient fertility evaluation. Some of the more effective meds out there for addressing hormone imbalances will boost pituitary function, if it's sagging. Clomiphene citrate is an old standby drug that may boost sperm counts and testosterone levels. Clomiphene is an off-label drug for men, but it has an excellent safety profile and has been studied extensively in male fertility, so I feel comfortable prescribing it for the appropriate person.

Procedures. As a reproductive surgeon specializing in microsurgery, I love to operate—but only on the right guy. And what I mean by that is a man with a varicocele—a varicose vein in the scrotum—which is the most common finding of a man with poor fertility (40 percent of men with fertility problems have varicoceles). With a varicocele, the veins bulge out around the testicle and overheat the sperm, causing poor sperm production and sluggish swimming. Luckily, the fix is pretty simple: I make a tiny incision in the groin and, using a surgical microscope, tie off all the bulgy veins to decompress and cool the scrotum. After about four months, the sperm counts and motility improve, and pregnancy rates typically jump 40 percent.

> ## MYTH: Testosterone Replacement Therapy Boosts Fertility
>
> It's shocking how many men I see who have been prescribed testosterone by another doctor to boost their sperm counts. Testosterone therapy will actually lower—or even completely wipe out—sperm production! Testosterone boosts sperm counts only when a man's body makes it itself. Sperm need high levels of naturally produced testosterone to grow and function properly. If you're trying to initiate a pregnancy and your T is low, I can prescribe medications to naturally increase your T production. But I can't give you testosterone—it's a very effective male birth control.

NEXT-LEVEL REPRODUCTION OPTIONS

These days there are so many reasons why a couple may need an assist from science: perhaps all else has failed for a man and woman, perhaps two men want to become dads to a biologically related child, or perhaps biological men want to affirm their female gender but retain their ability to have biologically related children. For all of the above, there is assisted reproduction. There are currently two leading ways of doing this (as well as several variations on the theme).

Intrauterine Insemination (IUI)

IUI is a fairly low-tech process that's good for a genetic male and genetic female who have mild barriers to conception, such as a woman having a tilted cervix or a man having low sperm counts (though, for IUI to have a chance, the man needs to have about three million swimming sperm in his ejaculation). For IUI, a reproductive gynecologist will track the genetic female's ovulation; when it is at its peak, the couple comes into the office, where the man masturbates into a collection cup and the lab processes the semen. The lab will put the semen into a special broth called sperm medium to give the sperm some sugar and other nutrients, which then gets inserted into the woman's cervix and pushes the sperm fluid directly into the uterus. The procedure takes about 30 seconds and is as uncomfortable as a routine pelvic exam. The partner then stays propped up for about 10 minutes to allow the sperm to move downhill and find an egg.

Success of pregnancy after IUI is less than 20 percent, but it can still be a great option when the couple has had a zero percent success rate through intercourse. IUI is a particularly useful alternative when the couple is not sexually active together, such as when the partner is a surrogate for a same-sex male couple. Likewise, if a man in a heterosexual couple has no sperm, the couple can use donor sperm. Since the procedure is usually less than $1,000, IUI is a cost-effective pathway to pregnancy. Some insurance plans cover fertility benefits including IUI, but many don't.

In Vitro Fertilization (IVF)

This is quite a bit more complex than IUI. In vitro fertilization is where the sperm from a man and the egg from the partner are put together to create an embryo (or, usually, multiple embryos). After a few days incubating, the best-quality embryos are either frozen for future pregnancies or implanted directly into the uterus of the woman who will be carrying the child. IVF opens up so many possibilities for all kinds of couples to achieve biologically related children, and it has excellent chances of pregnancy—upwards of 70 percent, in many cases. For same-sex male couples, IVF allows them to use their sperm and have a child with a surrogate. For transgender and non-binary couples, individuals assigned male at birth with the ability to provide sperm can choose to either impregnate their partner or use a surrogate to carry the pregnancy. IVF is a miracle treatment for many couples. But it comes at a price, and many insurance companies do not cover the treatment, which can easily cost tens of thousands of dollars. It can also be hard on a woman as she has to go through hormone therapies and procedures to retrieve the eggs to start the fertility process. But if you and your partner are able to achieve pregnancy through IVF, you will likely agree it was worth it.

A CALL TO ACTION There are studies that show that men who have difficulty initiating a pregnancy are at risk for a few health concerns, such as developing cancer later in life. There is no need to panic, but this does emphasize the importance of staying plugged in with your doctor and staying on top of getting annual checkups for the rest of your life. But then, that's good advice for all men.

ROB, 34

A Close Call

Rob was 34. He and his wife, Michelle, had a beautiful 2-year-old daughter, and they were trying for a second child. With their first child, Rob was 32, healthy, and they had no trouble getting pregnant. Michelle's ob/gyn suggested that Rob get a semen analysis. The results were troubling—his total sperm counts were 300,000, where they should have been over 40 million. The couple was now heading toward in vitro fertilization, and Michelle's reproductive endocrinologist suggested Rob see me to optimize his sperm counts. Rob was in excellent shape, fit, ran marathons, and worked a low-stress job in the tech sector. But I noticed he had a hard lump in his left testicle. I sent Rob immediately for an ultrasound. Sure enough, his left testicle had a large mass that would have to be removed. I told Rob to head to the sperm bank and deposit a few sperm samples, even though the numbers were low, so that they would at least have something if his sperm counts dropped further after surgery to remove his testicle. Within three days, Rob was in the operating room and I performed a radical orchiectomy, in which I removed his whole testicle and spermatic cord. The pathology showed Rob had testicular cancer (seminoma), which is aggressive but does not always need chemotherapy or radiation. And he recovered fine. Even more impressive, his sperm counts actually bounced back. Four months after his surgery, his sperm counts were in the five million range, and Michelle was pregnant a month later!

Preventing Pregnancy

You won the game. You have as many kids as you and your partner desire and now want to recreate, not procreate. Or you don't want to play the game and never want to play the game. Let's look at some options for male-centered birth control.

CONTRACEPTION OPTIONS

1. The Condom

Condoms have a long history. In Ancient Greece, men used goat and sheep bladders as wraps to prevent venereal disease and pregnancy. Ancient Egypt documented condom use—linen sheaths—likely not great at preventing pregnancy but employed mostly as fashion items as they were color-coded based on a man's social status. Modern condoms of rubber go back to the 1860s—once Charles Goodyear (yes, the tire guy) figured out how to make rubber more flexible, strong, and thin, the modern rubber was born. By the 1920s, latex came around, which was a more refined way to use rubber. Widespread condom use in the United States, however, didn't happen until the AIDS pandemic of the 1980s, when they became more popular as a way to save lives rather than prevent procreation.

Condoms today are further refined, made of synthetic materials to be more comfortable, stronger, and safer. But condoms still can fail as a birth control method. You have to know how to put them on properly. To be effective, they can't slip off during intercourse or break. The modern failure rate of a condom is less than 10 percent, so not bad. Many men complain that condoms decrease sensation and enjoyment of sex. But so does causing an unintentional pregnancy . . . so . . . your pick.

2. The Pullout

If you have perfect control of your ejaculatory threshold and can pull out prior to ejaculating in your partner's vagina every time, that's impressive. And also not likely. There are so many things wrong with the pullout method. First of all, very few men have that level of self-control. Second, men *can* begin emitting semen prior to full-on ejaculation. Bottom line: if you've successfully been pulling out for years and not initiated a pregnancy, you should get a sperm analysis as you may have fertility issues. Combining the pullout with tracking your partner's ovulation cycle is a bit sounder birth control but not one I would recommend.

3. The Snip

For any man who has decided it's time to close the factory and open the playground, he should have a vasectomy. A vasectomy basically blocks sperm from leaving the testicle, which is the only *nearly* 100 percent effective way for couples to ensure they don't get pregnant. It's a common procedure: I perform more than 400 vasectomies a year. These days, vasectomies are quick outpatient procedures—less than 15 minutes—usually performed under a local anesthetic. The incisions are usually so small, in fact, that many urologists, me included, perform a no-scalpel vasectomy, where we just poke a tiny hole in the skin and snake up the vas deferens through the hole. This procedure is certainly easier for a guy to get than it is for his female partner to undergo a permanent, nondrug sterilization such as a tubal ligation. For a woman, a tubal ligation represents an abdominal surgery, usually under general anesthetic, that has a pretty significant risk profile. Since our testicles, unlike our partners' ovaries, are external organs, access to the vas deferens is way easier. Also, the success rate of tubal ligation is not as high as vasectomy. Happily, couples who undergo a vasectomy report higher sex drives and more frequent sex than couples who use other forms of birth control. And if a guy and/or his partner change their minds, it's reversible.

Expect to have some bruising, swelling, and discomfort for a couple of days to a week. After about eight weeks, men should be cleared to have sex without another form of birth control. The more ejaculations a guy has in the weeks after his

How It Works: Vasectomy

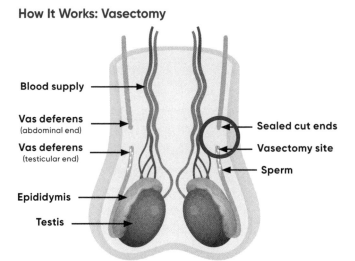

Semen is produced in the seminal vesicles and the prostate, then travels directly through the urethra. Sperm are made in the testicles and join the semen farther upstream, but they only make up about 1 percent of seminal fluid, which is why ejaculation doesn't change after a vasectomy. Snipping the vas deferens during a vasectomy simply traps sperm in the epididymis, where the body naturally breaks them down and recycles them.

procedure, the quicker he's shooting blanks. Of course, many men enjoy telling their partners that more sex is doctor's orders (I've had men ask me to write a prescription). A vasectomy does not change how much fluid comes out when a man ejaculates—semen comes from the prostate gland, and the seminal vesicles which are way downstream from the vasectomy site. I tell the man that the only way to tell if he's had a vasectomy would be by looking at his semen under a microscope. And a guy won't feel any different when he ejaculates (with one exception, postvasectomy pain syndrome, which I'll elaborate on), and he won't have any change in his erections. Testosterone levels also stay the same because the testosterone the testicles make circulates in the blood vessels, not the sperm ducts.

Vasectomy Reversals. Change your mind? I perform a lot of vasectomy reversals—men change their minds and sometimes change their partners. If you pick a capable surgeon with a high success rate, you have about a 90 percent chance of getting sperm back in the ejaculate. It's a two- to three-hour surgery under a general anesthetic where the doctor uses the surgical microscope to reconnect the vas deferens. The couple then has a good chance of conceiving spontaneously. Now if you don't want a reversal but would like to initiate a pregnancy, I can remove sperm from the testicle under a local anesthetic in a few minutes and give the sperm to your partner's reproductive specialist to make a baby with in vitro fertilization (IVF). This is also successful.

JACK, 40

The Genetic Vasectomy

Jack was a self-described player. He was 40 when he came to my clinic. He had been sexually active since he was a teenager with multiple partners, rarely used a condom, and had never initiated a pregnancy (that he knew about). He then found "the One." She was perfect, 32, healthy, no prior pregnancies, and with a green light from her ob/gyn that she was fertile. Jack was ready to settle down and be a dad. His wife made the appointment for Jack to see me. After my interview and physical exam with Jack where I could not feel his vas deferens, I asked him to provide a sperm sample. My lab ran the sample and showed me the results: no sperm! Fortunately for the couple, Jack had a genetic issue that blocked his sperm ducts but did not impair sperm production—he was essentially born with a vasectomy. I was able to surgically extract sperm, and the couple achieved pregnancy with assisted reproduction.

Still No Male Pill?!

But man, have we tried to make one. Clinical trials on male contraceptive pills date back to the 1980s. Stands to reason if a woman can take a pill, why can't a man? Scientists thought they had a good one 40 years ago—it was testosterone. When a man takes testosterone, his sperm counts go down. That's one of the more common causes of male infertility—a man is taking testosterone to boost his energy, muscle mass, sex drive, and erections. But pill forms of testosterone have traditionally been hard on the liver, and there are still plenty of guys who take testosterone and don't have sperm counts drop to zero. The failure rate with the T pill is unacceptable. But research continues, and we may in fact have a male birth control pill one day.

Rare—but Scary—Side Effects of the Snip

Rarely, complications happen as a result of a vasectomy. On the less-serious side, men can develop a hematoma, which is a painful collection of blood in the scrotum that can take weeks to resolve. Hematomas usually happen as a result of a guy getting back to full activity too soon. I always tell my men to wait a week or two, even before they get back to the gym. While also uncommon, a man can get an infection after a vasectomy. Tragically, I have also seen some devastating complications, where a man's testicle is injured or can even die from a vasectomy. This, thankfully, is *super* rare, but you have to know about this before you go through the procedure. There is also a very small percentage of men who develop long-term pain—months to years after the procedure—from a horrible condition called postvasectomy pain syndrome (PVPS). I've seen this condition in all types of men. There is also no way to predict whether someone will develop the condition before he undergoes the procedure. For that reason, I discourage men who already have pain in their scrotum from getting a vasectomy. If you've had a vasectomy and you're chronically in pain, see a urologist specializing in microsurgery so he or she can evaluate you.

PRECUM: A PREQUEL TO SEMEN

Yes, preejaculate fluid can get a woman pregnant, but it's very unlikely. Perhaps you're not quite ready for kids and are thinking of fertility in an entirely different way—how to make sure you *won't* get your partner pregnant. Preejaculate, or precum, as it's often called, is a sticky fluid secreted through a gland in the urethra that lubricates the urethra prior to ejaculation so the semen has a slick tube to travel through. There is no sperm in this fluid; what you learned in high school biology is wrong, sorry to say. But men start releasing semen (which, as you learned earlier, contains sperm) prior to ejaculation, so you can still get someone pregnant even if you think you're pulling out prior to the full finish.

Chapter Cheat Sheet

☐   The healthier you are, the more fertile you can be, if there are no underlying issues. Best way to improve your sperm counts? Eat, move, and sleep better!

☐   Fertility is both a male *and* female problem. Because it's so easy for guys to get checked, this should be the first step in attempting pregnancy.

☐   Sometimes, all it takes to conceive a child is a little help from a fertility specialist; there are several great therapies these days for men with impaired sperm function.

☐   If your baby-making days are behind you, consider a vasectomy as a safe permanent option.

07

LIFESTYLE

A Man's Guide to Living Well

I hate "wellness." Whatever you do, don't call this a wellness book. Let me clarify: I hate how wellness companies use this word to sell you everything from spa treatments to skin care to supplements. And what does *wellness* even mean? Yoga pants and aromatherapy? Stress reduction, eating well, sleeping, exercising, time with friends and family, sex, puppies, the smell of a baby's head? The word has lost all meaning. *Wellness* today refers to things many people don't think they can afford. Perhaps it's time to move on from this vague term and simply live well. **We have to stop commercializing the fundamentals of better living and simply eat, move, and sleep better. Living well, with the knowledge you learn in this book, won't cost you much money and won't require a lavender-infused sleep mask. (But it's**

totally cool to use one if it helps you sleep better.)

What I can live with are the words *healthy lifestyle*. In many ways, everything in this book falls under the umbrella of lifestyle. How do you want to style your life? Almost all aspects of men's health can be influenced by what we eat, how much we move, and how well we sleep.

Sleep is an interesting anomaly within medical science. It is a well-established and universal fact that our health depends on good sleep. Few things are as consequential to our physical and mental well-being. And yet there is very little research to help us define "good" sleep. One thing we do know is that sleep is highly individual. So here I'll cover what we *do* know and at least make you more aware of how well you are sleeping and motivate you to make changes, if necessary.

And since we've gone quite deep on the physical in this book, I'd like to highlight the importance of emotional health. Balancing the demands of your day job with taking more control of your health is not easy. I get it. Although I don't have any secrets, I do have lots of advice on how taking care of yourself will, in turn, make your day job better and make the people around you happier. So let's start by breaking down the monster topic of stress.

Managing Stress

Stress is a biological response that is as essential to survival as it is destructive. Animals get stressed, insects get stressed. Simple organisms stress about getting food, getting sex, or getting killed. My dog stresses about not getting his ears rubbed enough. Just like them, humans need stress to survive *and* thrive. At its worst, it causes stress hormones, blood pressure, and insulin levels to rise while causing dopamine, our reward and feel-good hormone, levels to drop. This physical response is designed to get us out of trouble, escape harm, or fight our way out of a situation. In a modern context, this response can drive us to perform better and be more productive. Except this drive often leads to wanting more, doing more, and achieving more, entering a cycle in which de-stressing is no longer an option. Financial, relationship, and health stress take men down. There is no medical cure for stress. It's a disease doctors struggle with. The neurochemical reason many men turn to alcohol or drugs to combat stress is that these drugs of abuse temporarily raise dopamine levels and thus make these men feel better, if only for a moment. But the more you drink or more drugs you do, the less dopamine reward you get and the more substances you need to take in. Everyone's threshold is different. Some men can enjoy a drink or two and not tend toward addiction; others will crave more and more and find themselves in an addictive spiral.

Learning how to harness stress is crucial. Get in the habit of acknowledging when you're having a stressful, day, week, month, or event. And acknowledge when it is time to let go of stress and the relentless drive to do, do, do. As a surgeon, I harness stress often. I can have intense periods of focus to make sure the man I'm operating on has a great surgical outcome. But in the moment, performing surgery is pretty freaking stressful—I literally have another man's life in my hands six to ten times a week.

REDUCING STRESS

Much of stress reduction lies in acknowledging that it is a part of life and harnessing it in healthier ways. Once you've learned to better acknowledge and harness stress, it's time to work on reducing it. First, allow yourself the time and space to decompress. Lucky for my dog, rubbing his ears causes my blood pressure to go down. Symbiosis. That's what you need as well—find a symbiotic organism where your coexistence de-stresses both of you. Your breakthrough moment will be when you get your dopamine from healthy sources like exercise, a satisfyingly healthy meal, or high-level intimacy with your partner. When you make that breakthrough, your life will change forever, for the better. The transition will happen. Here are a few more proven destressors:

Learn to Breathe

Ever wonder why we yawn? It's not exactly because our bodies need more oxygen—it's actually a complex physiologic reaction to cool brain temperatures. The bonus side effect of a good yawn is you get more oxygen deep in your lungs, stretch your breathing muscles, and relax your stress response. So yawning is literally a wake-up call that you're not breathing deeply enough. There was a cool study years ago that found that deep nose breathing significantly reduced yawning. Taking a series of three deep, expansive breaths—inhaling through your nose and exhaling through your mouth anytime you feel that pit of stress in your belly—will immediately reduce your stress level.

The Power of Meditation

I can't teach you to meditate in this book. It's complex, I'm not qualified, and the topic is a book in itself. But I will say that if you learn to meditate, you will have a powerful weapon in your antistress arsenal. Meditation engages the parasympathetic nervous system—this is your resting or relaxing nervous system. If you are able to engage the parasympathetic, the sympathetic stress system shuts down. Clinical studies support meditation's role as a reliever of chronic pain, depression, and a host of other psychiatric and physical disorders. A good place to start is with mindfulness meditation, which has been extensively studied: sound neuroscientific data shows it improves depressive symptoms, sharpens cognition, and can even boost your immune system. Mindfulness-based cognitive therapy (MBCT) is an accepted practice with certified instructors. You can locate certified instructors in your area, or, thanks to the advent of telehealth, you can often find practitioners who can instruct you via the Web. Most classes are eight weeks in length and vary in price but will be a great investment in yourself.

Unplug

Of course, I'm going to tell you to turn off your phone and technology to really decompress. I admit that as a physician who is essentially on call 24/7, unplugging is nearly impossible. But during those times I'm not on call for the emergency room or operating room, I carve out a half hour a day to put my phone and pager in another room, then decompress.

THE VICIOUS CYCLE: STRESS AND CHRONIC PAIN

Stress and chronic pain are evil twins that conspire to make you miserable. People who live with chronic pain, be it from migraines, back pain, gout, arthritis, whatever, experience flare-ups of their pain when stress levels spike. And the more stressed they get, the worse the pain becomes and the more miserable they feel. Chronic pain leads to poor work performance and status and, eventually, financial troubles. That leads to relationship troubles. Already undergoing health stress, these men now have the hat trick of animal stress fears: food, sex, survival.

If you have a chronic pain condition, naturally you should seek medical help. You may be prescribed pills; you may be told you need surgery. But before you rush into medication or surgery, step back for a moment: it's important to realize that traditional medical solutions will not address the root cause of your pain. If you're not receiving some kind of therapy—be it psychological or physical therapy/massage—to reduce stress, then you're not being fully treated. And I get it, it's not that simple. Before you get to that point, get the help you need, recalibrate what your priorities are, and come back twice as strong. In my practice, I see men with debilitating scrotal pain. I've seen airline pilots and surgeons with pain so severe they can't work. Sometimes I can offer them microsurgery to relieve their chronic pain, but I always treat them alongside my physical therapist and, if appropriate, psychotherapist colleagues as well. Multidisciplinary solutions often work best.

AVOID PEOPLE WHO TELL YOU THAT YOU NEED TO RELAX

I feel the same way about the phrase *You need to relax* as I do the word *wellness*. Don't tell someone who's stressed out to relax—such advice makes the situation worse. When a guy, obviously burdened to capacity, comes into my clinic, I start a conversation. I try to find out what he enjoys doing for himself. Whether it's vigorous exercise, listening to podcasts, or streaming content, I'm cool with it. I just want men to actively engage in stress reduction while doing their thing, and to be aware that this activity is downtime. If I am binge-watching a show, I'm usually cooking dinner or meal prepping while I'm watching—for me, that's the perfect amount of relaxation with a goal-oriented outcome. That's as relaxed as I ever get. But it works!

A CALL TO ACTION It's clear that the wheels have come off on your ability to manage stress when you get that gnawing pit in your stomach, as if you're about to speak in front of a crowd and have no speech, and you can't identify one stressful thing causing this feeling. This situation can be tricky to address. When stress begins to manifest physically, fall back on your support mechanisms. Talk with someone you trust, either an inner-circle friend or family member or even a professional. I find compartmentalizing severe stress works. Play the worst-case scenario game. You have a deadline, you miss a deadline. Do you get fired? Probably not. You get an extension and you grind it out. Usually, when your worst-case-scenario is your stress, you'll realize that whatever it is, it isn't that bad and you move on.

FACE FAILURE WITH GRACE

Men are particularly bad at admitting failure. To paraphrase Bruce Springsteen, there are only winners and losers; don't get caught on the wrong side of that line. Somewhere in our development, we got the message that failure is shameful. For us men, failure often equates to weakness, and we are particularly prone to harbor our failures internally, which leads to more stress. In men's health, if someone fails at a diet or exercise regimen, he is less likely to commit to another program. In relationships, failure holds men back from finding someone new. At work, failure prevents people from taking on new risks and new projects. Stop. Stop telling yourself failure is bad. Failure is inevitable if you put yourself out there. In fact, failure is a sign you are living a full life. I know it sounds like a bumper sticker, but *what you do when you recover from failure defines you*. Taste the pain of failure, embrace it, and be stronger, better, and faster next time.

BE VULNERABLE

It's good to be vulnerable. Men tend to shoulder burden differently than women. Men don't ask for help. Men don't cry. Of course, I'm making sweeping generalizations. Some men become puddles of vulnerability at the first sign of crisis. The point is, take a look at how you respond to crisis or sadness. Do you wall in or do you open up? If you have a partner you can confide in, do you reveal what worries you the most? Being vulnerable allows you to grow. So give up your stubbornness and open your mind. It took me decades to realize this, and I'm still working on being vulnerable. I'm a bull-headed surgeon who has figured out ways to do complicated, stressful tasks well, but that doesn't mean I know everything. I have to check myself in subjects I'm not so slick at and be vulnerable, be strong enough to admit I don't know and need help. Embrace that feeling—it's initially uncomfortable but ultimately empowering.

DO NOT FEAR THE BIG D

Men deal with depression differently than women and should approach dealing with it in different ways. Anytime a man comes into my office with signs of depression, I want to know, is it situational or chronic? Genetics plays a big role in rates of depression and how a man reacts to distressing circumstances. Things like financial stress, marital and family problems, or health issues can upset any of us. But for the most part, those are situational problems, which means the depression is both a temporary condition and can likely be treated with a lifestyle change, such as more exercise or better sleep. But when a man tells me he doesn't know or remember why he feels stressed or anxious, I'm more concerned. If he can't remember the last time he was happy, I worry. Many doctors will have patients fill out validated questionnaires to better characterize a person's risk of significant depression. Unfortunately, most men do not talk openly with other men about what's bugging them, and this could be one of the reasons why men have much higher substance abuse and suicide rates than women. These men often need professional help and therapy. **That said, I think *all* men can benefit from therapy if they can find a good therapist.** Your primary-care physician, if you have one, or your medical plan, if you have one, will offer recommendations for trusted therapists in your area who likely take your insurance. If you don't have a primary physician and don't have health insurance, get both! Until then, the American Psychiatric Association has a provider locator at finder.psychiatry.org that can get you started.

GETTING HIGH TO HANDLE THE LOWS

Cannabis is everywhere these days, in any form you desire. It's legal in so many states it's hard to keep track, and rarely a day goes by in Los Angeles that I don't end up inhaling a contact high on the street. Is this a good thing? Well, we don't have enough science on weed yet to know for sure. Weed advocates are quick to point out how safe it is compared to alcohol, but they are usually a little thin on evidence. While the medical community has studied alcohol for a hundred years, no such long-term studies have been conducted on pot.

We do know that cannabis is a great appetite stimulant, so people suffering from wasting diseases like terminal cancer, advanced AIDS, or muscular dystrophy and people on chemotherapy can benefit from ingesting it in edible or smoking form. Animal studies show cannabis improves inflammatory

Antidepressants

Why not put every depressed guy on antidepressants? In short, side effects. Most antidepressants are selective serotonin reuptake inhibitors (SSRIs). SSRIs are safe drugs with far fewer dangerous side effects than the older generation of antidepressants, but they do have several side effects that most guys don't want. SSRIs can stop, or dramatically delay, a man's ability to orgasm (in fact, I prescribe these drugs to men who ejaculate too soon). Imagine the frustration of a man on SSRI therapy who can have intercourse but can never finish. Some men also mention their libido decreases on SSRI therapy. So a depressed man has to make a choice—better mood, worse sexual function or worse mood, normal sex. I see a lot of men who have come to me because they want an alternative to an SSRI. There are SSRIs and antidepressant medications that are a little less guilty of knocking off your sex drive, so let your physician know you want the medication with the fewest sexual side effects. The two that work the best are bupropion (Wellbutrin) and duloxetine (Cymbalta).

bowel disease (IBD) symptoms. Placebo-controlled studies in humans don't show much of a benefit, but for men with IBD, medical marijuana may be worth a try. Cannabis may also be good for anxiety disorders, with a better side-effect profile than pharmaceutical anxiety pills. There is also compelling data showing that cannabis derivatives ease epilepsy seizures and that weed decreases eye pressure, which can help people with glaucoma. Like so many topics in health, weed consumption is not all good or not all bad. You have to ask yourself why you want to use it and what need are you trying to fill.

Mastering Sleep

We talk a lot about how important it is to eat well, yet we typically spend less than two hours a day eating. We talk about how important exercise is, yet we exercise only 30 minutes to an hour a day (if we're at the top of our game). So why not spend more time figuring out how to get better at something that actually takes up about a third of our day? From a medical standpoint, we are just starting to understand how complex sleep is—and how critical it is to good health. Despite the fact that sleep is a pillar of men's health—as important as eating right and moving regularly—the medical community has a lot of research to do to figure out causes and treatments for men who don't sleep well. Among the most important steps you can take to evaluate your own sleep quality is to keep a sleep journal. Also, keep your eyes and ears open for any new studies on sleep—they're coming out all the time—and educate yourself.

GOOD SLEEP IS ALL ABOUT QUANTITY *AND* QUALITY

The American Academy of Sleep Medicine recommends we get six to eight hours of sleep a night. We all have a circadian rhythm—the hormone-influenced sense of when we should be sleeping and when we should be awake—but it's not always in step with our life. Some people need a little more shut-eye, some a little less, and it's important to know your personal sweet spot. This was easy back before electricity and the internet, when we slept more or less from dusk until dawn. Now that we live in a 24-hour world, full of technology, it's more challenging than ever to get enough sleep. Note, however, that routinely sleeping *more* than eight hours could be a sign of a problem: thyroid disease, depression, or other mental health disorders. Bottom line: if you're not sleeping at least six hours a night consistently, you're ripping yourself off! All the gains you make with good nutrition and good exercise won't pay dividends if you're not catching enough z's.

POOR SLEEP IS THE SLIPPERY SLOPE

You'd be surprised how many health issues can arise if you are not sleeping well. Men who don't get into stage IV sleep don't restore testosterone levels. If a man isn't getting enough shut-eye, he can't recharge the pituitary gland, which is what governs the testicles' ability to make testosterone. Men's testosterone levels peak first thing in the morning and stay high for about four hours (from four to eight a.m. in a normal day-night cycle). If you aren't in deep sleep, in REM sleep, your pituitary gland can't signal the testicle to crank out T. Poor sleep causes depression, increases your risk of type II diabetes, and—oh yeah—makes you fat. Stress hormone levels go up in poor sleepers, which causes blood sugar levels to rise, insulin secretion to go up, and fat deposition to occur. It's crucial you either address poor sleep habits yourself or get professional help.

Poor sleep is probably the most common risk factor I see in otherwise normal men with low

testosterone. For those guys, when I check their blood testosterone levels, I also check luteinizing hormone (LH), which the pituitary gland secretes to goad the testicle into making more testosterone. If LH levels are low, I know the guy is stressed and not sleeping enough. Be aware that your primary-care physician usually won't check LH levels, and that's okay—it's a test that needs specialist interpretation.

SETTING THE SLEEP MOOD

Study after study has proven that a few basic conditions are conducive to better sleep:

DO

Sleep in a cool environment. Sleeping in a cooler room usually helps men get deeper sleep. The ideal temperature is 65 to 68 degrees Fahrenheit. As we sleep, our body temperature drops naturally, and cooling the room encourages our bodies to drift into deeper shut-eye.

Exercise regularly. Men who exercise more, whether at morning, noon, or night, sleep better. Figure out the best workout timing for you and keep as close to that time every day, if possible.

Offload stress before bed. One of the prime causes of sleep disorders is stress. Most of us men stress right before bed, when we begin to think we have too much to do and didn't get enough done that day. That's me, for sure. Learn how to offload your stress *before* bed. I find that making a mental checklist of what I accomplished that day and what I need to do in the future relaxes me. Writing the list down is helpful, too: it feels good to check off a box and move on. Of course, family stress, health stress, or financial stress are more complex. Just remember to acknowledge that the problems won't go away overnight. You owe it to yourself and your loved ones to take care of yourself, and sleep is critical to that.

DON'T

Have caffeine too close to bedtime. Caffeine takes roughly six hours to clear your bloodstream, depending on how much you drink and your individual metabolism. I'm sure you know someone who says he can drink coffee right before bed and fall asleep just fine (I'm one of those); such guys are less susceptible to caffeine-induced insomnia. Let them boast about that while you cut caffeine before bed and see if that makes a difference in your getting a solid night's sleep.

Drink alcohol at least two hours before bed. You may think booze makes you sleepy, but you're not actually sleeping—your brain is in suspended sleep rather than deep sleep. Aim to cut yourself off at least two hours before bedtime, and don't consume more than two drinks at a sitting. It doesn't matter what you drink—beer, wine, or hard booze—the alcohol in all of them prevents sound sleep.

Let exercise interfere with sleep. There is no science that says exercising too close to bedtime is bad or good—the effects are individual, and you have to run your own experiment. Some men feel that working out before sleep helps them fall asleep faster and sleep longer and deeper. But others feel it keeps them wired long into the night. Both experiences are real, so it's important to know which category you fall into. Keep a sleep and exercise log to see whether you sleep better after a challenging evening workout or one completed earlier in the day. There are plenty of sleep-tracking apps if you're tech-minded. Or you can simply keep a pen and paper on your nightstand: write down when you exercised, when you went to bed, and ultimately how well you slept. After a week or so, you'll follow the trend.

The Four Stages of Sleep

Specialists divide sleep into four stages to better characterize and understand how we sleep. Different activities happen in these four stages.

- **Stage I.** You're still pretty awake, relaxing, although your mind is swirling. You're usually in stage I for 5 or 10 minutes.

- **Stage II.** You display the first signs of physiologic sleep, where body temperature and heart rate drop. This is drowsy sleep and lasts 10 to 20 minutes.

- **Stage III.** You're unconscious, your blood pressure and temperature drop further, and you're officially asleep. Stage III in some ways is the deepest sleep you'll get all night.

- **Stage IV.** Your unconscious brain activity skyrockets. This is dream or rapid eye movement (REM) sleep, where the body fully relaxes and the eyes rapidly move as your brain activity goes up. In REM sleep, the brain pretty much goes rogue and makes you dream about flying unicorns and giving speeches dressed only in your underwear. REM sleep is also when hormone levels rebalance for the next day.

SOME SLEEP ISSUES REQUIRE A SPECIALIST

Turning to your primary doctor for sleep advice is a good start. Your physician can definitely help you determine if you have a sleep *disorder* or if you simply have poor sleep habits. But your doctor will also know when it's time to refer you to a sleep center. True sleep disorders are chronic medical conditions that can even cause early death. First figure out whether you have trouble *falling* asleep or *staying* asleep. Then, to unearth what exactly is going on, a sleep specialist will often have you undergo an overnight sleep study to determine which medical—or possibly surgical—intervention makes sense. The two most common issues that warrant seeing a sleep specialist are:

Snoring, which can be a sign you're never getting into deep REM sleep in the first place.

Sleep apnea, a condition in which you stop breathing when asleep. If your partner sees you stop breathing for a few seconds and then kick back in, that's apnea, and you need to see a specialist. There are fantastic therapies for sleep apnea. One is CPAP, which stands for continuous positive airway pressure. A CPAP is a medical device you wear like a mask that gently puffs air into your lungs to keep your airway open as you sleep. It's the best nonsurgical treatment we have for apnea.

There's another reason you may have sleep challenges, and it's one that doesn't have to be addressed by a sleep specialist: if you have to pee a lot at night, you may have a condition known as nocturia, which can disrupt your sleep. Start with simple solutions like avoiding alcohol a few hours before you go to bed and limiting all fluids to two hours before. An enlarged prostate can make you get up to urinate often (see page 67), but this isn't the only cause. Men with heart failure pee more at night because the fluid buildup in their legs gets back to their kidneys faster when they're lying down and not fighting gravity. Men with diabetes go more frequently because the high blood sugar acts like a diuretic. And men taking diuretics for high blood pressure also pee more, by design. If you have to take diuretic medications, take them as far away from bedtime as you can so that you pee off the excess fluid before bed.

SAFE SLEEP SUPPLEMENTS

By now, you know that I'm not a big fan of supplements, unless there is great data to support their use. But when it comes to sleep, a few supplements have some decent studies. And since none of these can harm you if taken according to the label, even if they make you *think* they're helping you sleep, by all means take them.

Melatonin. Melatonin is the day-night hormone that regulates our circadian rhythms and it is perhaps the hottest natural sleep supplement out there. Studies have shown that taking between 3 and 10 milligrams of melatonin helps improve sleep in men who work night shifts. This makes sense: if you work nights, your circadian rhythm is deranged, and melatonin may help trick your brain into thinking three p.m. is three a.m. And this means it can also be effective for those with less-disruptive sleep schedules. People often tout this drug as a cure for jet lag, but it hasn't quite stood up to clinical trials yet. That said, I know a lot of physician friends who swear by it.

Valerian root. *Valeriana officinalis* is a flowering plant native to Asia and Europe. Traditional medicine has used valerian root for thousands of years for many purposes, to alleviate everything from anxiety to headaches to heart palpitations. Modern medicine has studied the root as a sleep aid. Studies show valerian root helps people fall asleep faster and sleep deeper (at doses of 300 to 900 milligrams). One solid study even showed it can work as well as a prescription sleep drug, so it's definitely worth a try before taking a prescription medication. Chemicals in valerian appear to bind to the same brain receptors as benzodiazepines like diazepam (Valium) or alprazolam (Xanax). For that reason, don't combine valerian root with other sleep medications or alcohol as it may work too well and knock you way out.

Magnesium. I'm reading more and more about magnesium these days—but I'm not sure it works for sleep quite like people say. A few good studies in the medical literature suggest magnesium supplements improve sleep in people who have low magnesium levels. But supersizing your magnesium load doesn't make you sleep better. Two fantastic sources of magnesium are green leafy vegetables and tree nuts, two of my go-to foods for better men's health. So guess what? I'm telling you to eat more green leafy vegetables and nuts and save your money on magnesium pills. Now if you are sleeping poorly and constipated, adding magnesium supplements, around 300 milligrams a day, can help slick up the bowels. Just don't pop the magnesium on a red-eye if you're in a window seat. You can take magnesium in a tablet, often combined with calcium, or you can take it as a liquid in the form of magnesium citrate.

Chamomile. Commonly found in tea, this is another "can't hurt, might help" for me. Chamomile is a flower in the daisy family that has been used in traditional medicine for thousands of years. Reports of medicinal chamomile use go back to ancient Rome, where its extract treated everything from seasonal allergies to menstrual cramps to, yes, sleep. There are many active chemicals in chamomile, but the one most studied is apigenin. Apigenin is soluble only in alcohol or oil, so if you want to take chamomile, you should take it as an extract of at least 1.2 percent. Some studies show it can help people over 65 get to sleep faster, but other studies say it's bunk. Most likely, the formulation matters. People taking an oil or extract will get more active ingredient, whereas people drinking a water-based tea may not be getting the effective level of apigenin. But perhaps the very act of making some hot, noncaffeinated tea before bed relaxes you and simply allows you to decompress. Either way, if it works for you, go for it. Be careful not to drink too much liquid too close to bedtime.

 PROCEED WITH CAUTION
Prescription Sleep Drugs

Prescription sleep medication has a long way to go. Drugs like clonazepam (Klonopin), zolpidem (Ambien), and others *will* help you fall asleep, but you'll never enter deep sleep, which is the most important part of the sleep cycle. Sometimes these drugs help you get a little shut-eye in a pinch—say, on an overnight flight—but taking them every day will turn you into a zombie. These drugs actually have the same effect alcohol does. The drug you *really* want to avoid is trazodone (Desyrel). Trazodone can cause priapism, a surgical emergency where the penis gets an erection that doesn't go away. A priapism lasting more than four hours can cause irreversible damage to normal erectile tissue: truly too much of a good thing. It's rare, and many docs don't know that trazodone causes priapism, but I've seen a lot of trazodone priapism, and any urologist will tell you it's a dangerous drug.

MOHAMMED, 34

Sleep Made the Difference

Mohammed was tired. Really tired. He was trying to make partner in his cutthroat law firm. He came to me with his wife and with dark circles under his eyes. Mohammed was sleeping, at best, 4 hours a night and working 16-hour days. He was 34 going on 60, *and* the couple was trying to have a baby. He didn't exercise. He ate fast food whenever he could, usually in his car on the way to work and on the way home late at night. His blood work showed testosterone levels were low for his age but not as bad as I would have imagined given how much stress he was under. What was shocking was his sperm counts. I found *five* sperm in his entire semen sample—normally men should have over 40 million sperm in each ejaculate. Five sperm. No wonder the couple couldn't get pregnant. I performed a full reproductive workup, including genetic tests to make sure he didn't have a biologic reason for his low sperm counts, and this all came back normal. So I prescribed he sleep at least 6 hours a night, stop consuming fast food, start eating a whole-food diet, and, if he could manage, get 30 minutes of exercise each day. Well, he didn't eat better or start exercising, but he did start sleeping closer to 8 hours a night. Three months later, his sperm counts crept into the five million range. The couple became pregnant a month later. Eating right, exercising, and sleeping well are all important, but at least focus on one. Mohammed has since become a dad, made partner, and is eating, moving, *and* sleeping better. And most important, he's happy.

TO NAP OR NOT

There is good science that supports the notion that a nap can improve your productivity. I think naps are like coffee: if they work for you, go for it; if they don't, don't feel obligated to start. I can't nap to save my life, so I'm not going to adopt the habit. When I was in surgical training, I noticed that some of my fellow residents could take a nap after being up all night, then be okay to work *another* full day. If I did that, I'd feel worse. I always found a five-minute shower beats a two-hour nap to help me grind out another 12 hours.

Look Good, Feel Good

Of course men are vain. We don't like to admit it, but most of us like to look good. We want nice hair, nice skin, and a nice physique, and we hope we age well. And yet, in general, the beauty market and the medical cosmetic market cater mostly toward women. Thankfully, societal norms are changing and men are increasingly more comfortable with the cosmetic side of self-care.

AGING GRACEFULLY

Women have long taken the lead in aging slowly and keeping up youthful appearances. Many men have this idea that they shouldn't care about how they look and age. But that doesn't have to be true, and in recent years, this perception has been changing. Cosmetic companies have begun marketing antiaging serums and skin-care products to men. Cosmetic dermatology also has turned its eye toward men. My general philosophy is, whatever you want to do to feel better about yourself, whether inside or out, is okay by me. If you are eating a great diet, exercising at the top of your game, and sleeping six hours plus, why not take it to the next level?

A GUIDE TO HAIR GROWTH

For many men, their hair defines them—it may even be, in their opinion, their best feature. If they start to bald, it can be devastating. One word of advice if you know someone who is losing his hair: do not tell him you'll love him anyway. That's not exactly what he wants to hear. Listen first, see what ideas he may have for addressing the problem, then support him whether he decides to shave it or treat it. Here's what is available for men losing their hair.

Medication

Three types of medications effectively prevent hair loss and restore some regrowth: minoxidil (Rogaine), dutasteride (Avodart), and finasteride (Propecia). Minoxidil at 2 to 5 percent concentration opens up blood vessels in the scalp to nourish the hair follicle. There are essentially no side effects to minoxidil. It's a gel or cream applied directly to the scalp and hair follicle so it doesn't get significantly absorbed into the bloodstream. Dutasteride and finasteride are both 5-alpha reductase inhibitors, or hormone blockers, that inhibit a testosterone hormone (dihydrotestosterone, or DHT) that leads to increased hair loss. Dutasteride and finasteride have a couple of unfortunate side effects. Some men who take these drugs report a drop in sex drive. Even less common is growth of breast tissue (gynecomastia). And since finasteride and dutasteride are hormone blockers, new dads should be careful with finasteride and wash their hands before they touch their babies.

Finasteride's Rare Side Effect

One cautionary word about finasteride: there is something called post-finasteride syndrome (PFS), which is a poorly understood but devastating condition. Imagine being 19 and starting to lose your hair. You go online, purchase finasteride, and start taking it. Weeks later, you stop waking up with erections or you lose your desire for sex. You ask Dr. Google what's up, and there's ten million hits on PFS. Unfortunately, there is no FDA-approved treatment for PFS. Stopping the medication works most of the time, but a small percentage of men never recover normal sexual function. I believe finasteride is a very good and safe drug, but I do counsel all my men on this rare side effect. All drugs have risks.

Hair Transplant

A hair transplant remains the gold standard for hair restoration. It's expensive, but it works. The concept is simple, although execution requires a very skilled surgeon. The surgeon will harvest hair follicles from the hairline you still have, then transplant them into the areas where you've lost hair. It then takes quite a while to grow, so you have to be okay with either being out of the public eye for a while or okay with people knowing you've had the procedure. If you have a great surgeon, eventually your hair will look pretty close to natural. This is why it's really, really important to shop around for a board-certified plastic surgeon or dermatologist who *specializes* in hair restoration. The American Society of Plastic Surgeons has a surgeon locator at find .plasticsurgery.org that can point you to a board-certified surgeon specializing in hair transplant. Be warned that a lot of less-reputable outfits out there will take your money and leave you looking worse.

Hair Growth Scams

Platelet-rich plasma (PRP) therapy and laser therapy are two other well-known hair replacement options, but they are long shots at best. PRP therapy is a procedure in which plasma from your blood—which typically promotes healing—is injected into your scalp to stimulate hair growth. PRP has unproven applications in orthopedics to improve joint healing and in sexual medicine to improve erectile function. For hair loss, there is some data to suggest it *may* help, but nothing too convincing.

Laser therapy is used in so many branches of medicine it's no surprise there's a market in hair restoration. The concept is simple: aim a laser at the scalp to generate a tissue reaction and shock the hair follicle into restarting hair growth. It's safe, but there is no compelling high-level medical research that supports the practice. The only way I would suggest these fringe therapies is under the supervision of a top dermatologist or plastic surgeon. Whatever you do, don't buy a hair laser out of an airline magazine or online.

IS HUMAN GROWTH HORMONE (HGH) A FOUNTAIN OF YOUTH?

HGH is an FDA-approved therapy for prepubescent children who are not reaching their ideal heights. Pediatric endocrinologists prescribe it legally and on label. Every other physician? Not so much. But its *off*-label use is what people talk about. I see men in my clinic who swear it helps them recover from workouts faster and makes them feel more vital. In fact, some call it a fountain of youth, since HGH is something our bodies actually produce a ton of when we're young (but doesn't seem to work so well when we're older). And I'm cool with that—as long as these guys understand that they may be paying a lot of cash for a placebo effect. You see, the data on HGH simply doesn't stand up to randomized, placebo-controlled scrutiny. Despite that dearth of data, there are hundreds, if not thousands, of clinics nationwide selling HGH for hundreds, if not thousands, of dollars a month. HGH is probably pretty safe—though it can cause joint pain and fluid retention—even if it doesn't work.

SMOOTH SKIN FOR HIM

For years, cosmetic dermatology—and related marketing machines—focused on keeping women's faces looking younger. Men get wrinkles in their faces, too, but society usually gives us men a pass as we age, gray, and wrinkle—apparently, men get more *distinguished*-looking. (Thank goodness, many women these days are breaking the stereotype cycle and aging gray and beautifully.) But here's the thing: guys should be able to consider cosmetic dermatology, too, if it will make them feel better about themselves (even if they do need to call it Brotox). If a guy wants to flatten his brow and crow's feet, he should. Botox is a biologic toxin that paralyzes the nerves in our facial muscles to flatten out the skin on top; one injection can last for four to six months and provide a less-wrinkled appearance. It is an easy procedure, there are no known long-term medical side effects, and it can be repeated for years. There are, in fact, all kinds of naturally derived fillers that can be injected into deep wrinkles in the face to soften a man's appearance. They are safe, effective, and totally up to you.

Scrotox (Yes, It's What It Sounds Like)

Yes, scrotox is a thing: the injection of Botox with the goal of achieving a saggier scrotum. Why would anyone want this? Turns out, not all scrotums are the same. Some men have a very tight scrotum, and their testicles don't hang down at all—it's as if they were always sitting in a cold lake. This can be very uncomfortable and, in some circles, unsightly. The scrotum has a bunch of muscles in it that rise and fall, usually in response to temperature changes. Injecting Botox into the scrotum will relax those muscles and let the testicles hang lower. This treatment is safe, effective, and totally up to you.

THE SUN CONUNDRUM

One of the biggest risk-versus-reward questions in men's health is sun exposure. In fair-skinned guys, prolonged exposure to sunlight even with adequate sunscreen causes skin cancer. However, we also know that sunlight is good for us because it increases vitamin D levels (low vitamin D levels cause bone loss, depression, infertility, immune system dysfunction, and a host of other bad stuff). Now, here's where things get tricky: we doctors believe vitamin D supplements don't work as well as sunlight in improving vitamin D deficiency, but we're not sure. It's also probably not true that sunscreen blocks vitamin D production and causes vitamin D deficiency. (There are no good studies showing a link between sunscreen and D deficiency; however, the newer sunscreens with sun-protection factors of 50 and above have not been studied and may in fact block vitamin D production from sunlight.) That said, skin cancer is no joke, and it's all too common. If I were your dermatologist, I would tell you to always cover up in

STUART, 37

Talk It Out

Stuart came to me because he was having trouble having an orgasm. He is 37, an entertainment agent, has an A-list clientele that he's built up over the last 15 years through brutal work hours. His primary physician started him on sertraline, an antidepressant and anxiety reducer, because he couldn't stop worrying about everything—the next contract, getting his kid into the swanky private school, his mom's declining health. He worked out with a trainer 4 days a week and was in perfect physical shape. He ate healthfully and slept okay (6 or 7 hours but not the most restful). The sertraline really helped calm his anxiety, but now he was stressed that he couldn't orgasm. His wife was taking it personally, and they had been avoiding intimacy because Stuart was a goal-oriented overachiever. The goal of sex is to finish, after all, at least in his mind. His workup was normal, vital signs perfect, blood tests all normal. How do I fix this guy? His lack of orgasm is a known side effect of antidepressants, and yet the medication was doing him a lot of good. I had no medical option. Therapy. Stuart began working with a sex therapist who counseled him to stop thinking about orgasm as necessary to enjoy sex. Disassociating the finish from the act helped him relax and start enjoying sex again, even if every encounter didn't end with his orgasm. Sometimes, we have to adjust what we are used to doing to grow as men.

the sun to prevent skin cancer and premature aging skin. That is good *medical* advice.

But as a men's health specialist practicing in sunny Southern California, I see a lot of guys who love to be out in the sun. It makes them happy. And I want them to be happy. But I don't want them to develop skin cancer. A commonsense rule is to limit sun exposure to unprotected skin to less than 15 minutes a day. And never, ever, ever get a sunburn—that's where all the bad stuff happens. Applying sunblock with an SPF of 15 to 30, especially on the face, prevents burning, reduces aging, and lowers skin cancer risk while still allowing the sunlight to make vitamin D. And while many dark-skinned men think they have a lower skin cancer risk than fair-skinned folks, it's nowhere near zero, so I give them the same advice. The most aggressive skin cancer, melanoma, may be harder to detect in darker skin, as the cancerous lesions are dark in color as well. Every man should get a mole check—a full body examination every year and point out any changes in mole size or consistency to their doctors.

Chapter Cheat Sheet

☐ Stress is essential to life. Embrace your stress to become stronger.

☐ You're nothing if you're not sleeping; 6 to 8 hours is ideal.

☐ Love how you look or get the help you need to look the way you want.

☐ Get some sun and some vitamin D to avoid the other big "D": depression.

☐ Be proactive on hair loss. If you're starting to thin, get help early on.

☐ It's okay to be vain—men can feel good about looking good, too.

SUPPLEMENT ROUNDUP

Here are the evidence-based supplements that you've seen throughout the book:

NAME	DOSE	USE	FOUND IN NATURE?
B-complex vitamins	See label	Energy, metabolism	Meat, vegetables
Chamomile	1.2% extract, see label	Sleep	Chamomile flower
Coenzyme Q10	200 mg/day	Immune health, Fertility	Fish, meats, grains
Creatine	Varies by goals (see page 145)	Athletic health	Meat, fish
Fish oil	1000 mg/day	Fertility	Oily fish like salmon
Folic acid	400 mg/day	Fertility	Greens, beans
Korean ginseng	600-900 mg/day	Erectile health	Ginseng root
L-arginine	500-3000 mg/day	Erectile health, athletic health	Meats, grains
L-carnitine	1,000mg/day	Fertility	meats
L-citrulline	500-3000 mg/day	Erectile health, athletic health	watermelon
Maca	Varies by label	Erectile health	Maca root
Melatonin	3-10 mg at bedtime	Sleep	Tart cherries, grains, tree nuts
Psyllium husk	See label	Gut health	Psyllium plant
Quercetin	See label	To improve BPH symptoms (see page 67)	Green tea, onions, buckwheat, many other plants
Selenium	80 mcg/day	Fertility	Tree nuts, fish, meat, grains
Valerian root	300-900 mg/day	Sleep	Valerian root
Vitamin C	250-500 mg/day	Immune health, fertility	Citrus, peppers, broccoli
Vitamin D	2,000 units/day	Immune health, bone health	Sunlight, meat
Zinc	75 mg/day	Immune health	Meat, greens, mushrooms

NOW IT'S UP TO YOU

Life is complicated, messy, stressful, and, at times, overwhelming. Solid health care is not. The pillars of men's health will remain the same. **Whatever you take from this book, I want you to fall back on the three pillars of eat, move, and sleep to organize your health.**

Where is men's health going? We've come a long way since the little blue pill landed on the market in 1998. Men are seeking out healthcare more often. There is heightened awareness of men's health issues in the media and marketplace. There are men's health organizations like Movember and TrueNorth Health Foundation that are raising millions of dollars to improve mental and cancer health for men. Maybe I'm so deep into it that I'm seeing more progress than there is, but I am feeling a true shift in how men engage the healthcare community. Men are seeking access to care and are getting screened for prostate and colon cancer in higher numbers.

What I see for the future of health technology is a pipeline of products that will monitor health status remotely. Imagine having a noninvasive way to monitor key blood work like blood sugar, thyroid, cholesterol, and testosterone levels so that your numbers will be waiting for you when you see your doctor. Imagine gathering more genetic information to predict how you will respond to a drug before your doctor prescribes it.

I am also superoptimistic that men's health will move from a niche service reserved for affluent men to an expansive healthcare offering that *all* men can afford and will have access to. At UCLA, we have many initiatives to provide high-quality men's healthcare to men of all socioeconomic levels. Not only are we changing the diversity of access to care, but we are also changing the diversity of practitioners in men's health. We enthusiastically recruit underrepresented minorities to train at UCLA from the undergraduate level through medical school, residency, and post residency fellowships. The future of men's health, as I see it, will be full of technological advances and social advances to make all men feel comfortable engaging with the healthcare system.

ACKNOWLEDGMENTS

I must thank Kitty Cowles, my agent, who convinced me I had the time (hah!) and expertise to pull this book off. Will Cockrell, my co-author, organized my thoughts, musings, and writing into the book in your hands. Artisan Books: my publisher, Lia Ronnen, my fantastic editors, Shoshana Gutmajer and Elise Ramsbottom, and the entire team, specifically, Suet Chong, Carson Lombardi, Zach Greenwald, Nancy Murray, Allison McGeehon, Theresa Collier, Amy Kattan Michelson, Patrick Thedinga, and Paula Brisco; they created a platform and gave me a voice to change the lives of men for the better through simple actions and sound guidance from their physicians. Translating a physician's medical jargon and shorthand into something readable is a tall order that requires many eyes and pens to get right.

To the men I've treated, I thank you for your trust, for teaching me, and for inspiring me to bring it every day, for every case.

To the mentors, Drs. Richard Williams, Jay Sandlow, Andy Meacham, and Larry Lipshultz, and to Dr. Mark Litwin, my mentor and chair: I am forever grateful for your wisdom and guidance.

To my trainees: you don't get it now, but when you become the trainer, you will feel the profound pride that the best in you lives on in those you train.

To my wife, Krista, and my children, Willem and Nelson: thanks for sharing me; medicine is a jealous mistress. You inspire me to be better and live better, and you bring me the joy I wish all men can experience.

To my parents, Sue and Dean: From your Iowa farm upbringings, you instilled in me the values of hard work and honesty. From your international wanderlust, you taught me to love the world and all its inhabitants.

To my brother: the real scientist in the family. I'll pay my way to Stockholm to watch you accept your prize.

To Kellie: for keeping my professional life organized and believing in the dream.

To Walt and Heide: for welcoming me into the family and letting me con your daughter into marrying me.

To Dr. Dyvon Walker: for your tireless research to help me fill in the blanks and for your life story— you are entering a noble profession where you will make impactful contributions.

To Uri Herscher, thank you for your wisdom, your counsel, your advice, and your friendship. Your life's work gives me hope the world is headed for better times.

And to Archibald Joseph: six years with you was better than a lifetime without you.

INDEX

JESSE N. MILLS, MD, is a leading expert in the field of men's health and sexual and reproductive medicine. He is a graduate of the University of Iowa Carver College of Medicine, trained in general surgery and urology at the University of Colorado, and completed a fellowship in male reproductive medicine and microsurgery at Baylor College of Medicine. He has had a medical practice devoted solely to men's health since 2008. He founded the first comprehensive men's clinic in Colorado, the Center for Men's Health at TUCC, in 2013, and founded the Men's Clinic at UCLA, where he currently serves as director, in 2016. In his role with UCLA Health, Dr. Mills serves as a medical consultant to the LA Lakers and LA Dodgers. He is also on the faculty of the David Geffen School of Medicine at UCLA and is a professor of urology at UCLA. He sees over three thousand new patients yearly for conditions as diverse as low testosterone, erectile dysfunction, male infertility, and Peyronie's Disease and lectures internationally on men's health topics. He has authored multiple peer-reviewed scientific papers and book chapters that may cure the average reader of insomnia. He lives in Los Angeles with his wife of nearly 30 years. They spend their free time cooking healthy, internationally inspired meals, exercising, and reading.